Med express

overcoming insomnia

TRIDENT
REFERENCE PUBLISHING

NOTE
This publication is intended to provide reference information for the reader on the covered subject. It is not intended to replace personalized medical diagnosis, counseling, and treatment from a doctor or other healthcare professional.
Before taking any form of treatment you should always consult your physician or medical practitioner.
The publisher and authors disclaim any liability, loss, injury or damage incurred as a consequence, directly or indirectly, of the use and application of the contents of this book.

Published by:
Trident Reference Publishing
801 12th Avenue South, Suite 400
Naples, Fl 34102 USA
Phone: + 1 239 649 7077
Email: sales@trident-international.com
Website: www.trident-international.com

Overcoming Insomnia

Publisher
Simon St. John Bailey

Editor-in-chief
Isabel Toyos

Art Director
Aline Talavera

Photos
© Trident Reference Publishing, © Getty Images,
© Jupiter Images, © Planstock, © J. Alonso

Includes index
ISBN 1582799687 (hc)
UPC 615269996874 (hc)
ISBN 1582799563 (pbk)
UPC 615269995631 (pbk)

2005 Edition
Printed in USA

overcoming insomnia

4 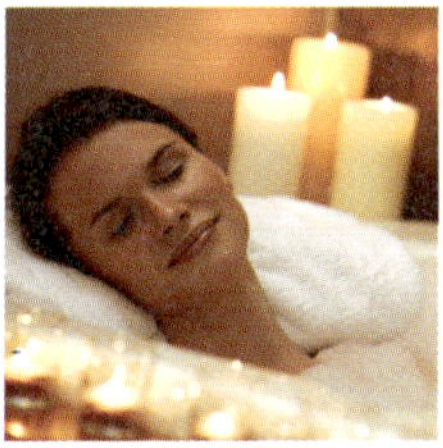 Introduction

12 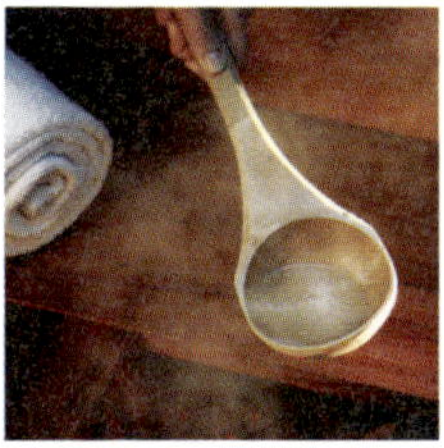 Complementary Therapies

40 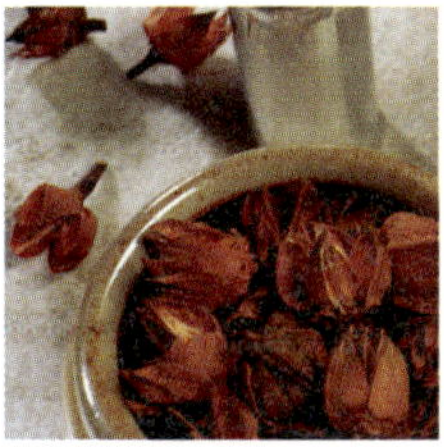 Natural Herb Remedies

50 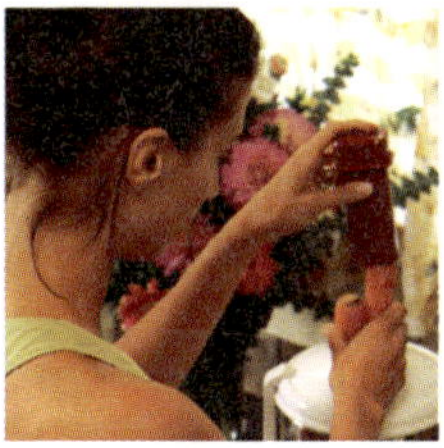 Healing Foods

What is insomnia?

Sleep is one of the most important and natural functions that human beings need on a daily basis. It is also one of the most vulnerable functions because of the physical and outside factors that prevent us from resting. One out of three Occidental people suffers from insomnia.

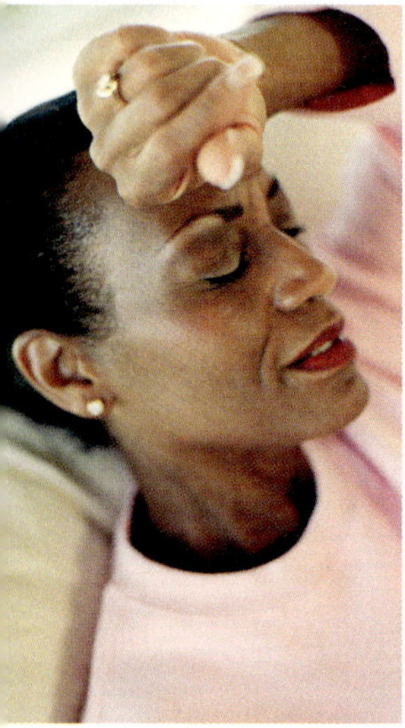

✚ Sleep helps the mind and body to rejuvenate and restore energy used during the day, to help keep us active and alert during our daily activities.

While we sleep we enter a periodic state of rest during which our consciousness of the world is suspended, allowing our bodies to rest up. Our brains have a number of functions, structures and "sleep centers" that regulate the cycle of sleep and wakefulness. At the same time, our bodies produce substances that when released into the blood stream, make us sleepy. When this process is altered –by stress, worries, disorders and physical ailments– we may suffer from insomnia.

THERE ARE THREE TYPES OF INSOMNIA

- **Acute/Transient Insomnia.** Lasts from one night to a few days. It is often caused by temporary changes in our lives such as, travelling, changes in schedule, worries or arguments.

- **Light Insomnia.** It is caused by some illnesses and physical disorder, or by periods of circumstantial stress. Lasts no longer than three weeks.

■ **Chronic Insomnia.** For specialists, this is a real sleep disorder. Occurs on most nights, causing anguish and lasts a month or more (sometimes years). According to the stages of sleep in which appears, insomnia can be classified as:

- **Initial.** Difficulty falling asleep; this is the most common symptom.
- **Intermittent.** Waking frequently during the night and having difficulty falling back to sleep.
- **Terminal.** Waking more than normal and not being able to fall back to sleep.

SLEEPING DISORDERS

- *When you don't sleep, or fail to pass through any stages of the sleep cycle.*
- *When you have difficulty reaching stages III and IV in the sleep cycle, making you sleep poorly and suffer from diurnal somnolence.*
- *When you sleep you can't reach REM, the stage in which you dream and which is necessary for the release of tensions and anxiety. Lack of REM can cause restlessness and emotional instability.*
- *When you frequently wake during the night, you feel fatigued as if you didn't rest.*

WHAT ARE THE STAGES OF SLEEP?

The body enters different stages of sleep ranging from light sleep to a deep sleep state. The diagram illustrates a normal sleep pattern for young adults.

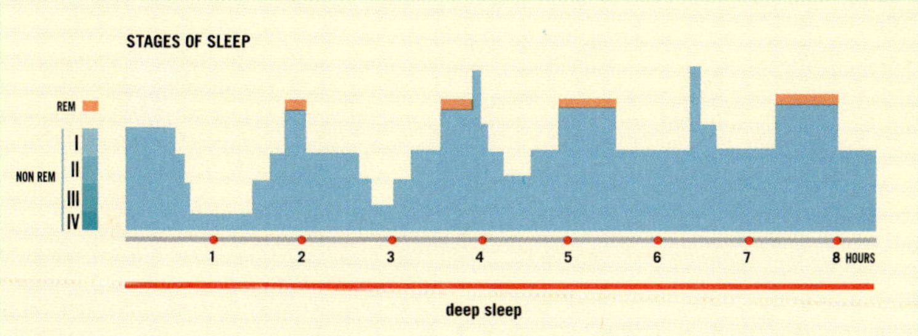

Phase I
When you fall asleep, you enter a light sleep and your brain continues to be stimulated.

Phase II
The brain waves become slower and the nervous system blocks our ability to read sensory information, that helps us sleep. This type of sleep helps to rejuvenate our bodies, but is not enough to rest completely.

Phase III
The brain waves become even slower, inducing a deeper sleep. This is an essential stage to fully rest.

Phase IV
Deep sleep is the most intense stage of sleep, with brain waves slowing to the maximum. It is a fundamental stage to restore the body and the mental state.

What causes insomnia?

Trying to go to sleep when you are tired and not being able to fall asleep can be torture. You don't need to have chronic insomnia to want to find tips on how to get a restful night of sleep. There are things you can do to help even slight sleeping disorders, even if you are anxious and upset and can't "catch a wink of sleep" during the course of a single night.

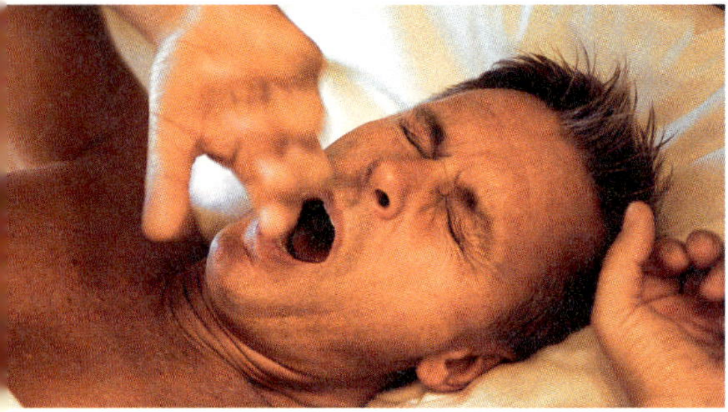

There are a number of factors that may cause you to experience insomnia. Some include:

- **Stress.** When you are anguished by personal problems and depression.
- **Lifestyle factors.** Changes in sleep schedules, staying up all night, problems at work, jet lag, partying, over-long naps and erratic hours.
- **Environment factors** Noise, uncomfortable bed, soft mattress, hard

KEEP A SLEEP DIARY

Keeping track of your daily sleep habits in a diary can help you recognize what factors and/or habits prevent you from getting a restful night of sleep. In the morning, jot down what time you went to bed the night before, how long it took you to fall asleep, if you woke up during the night, what you thought about or if you were worried before going to bed and what you ate at dinner. After 15 days you will have a chart of your common habits and be able to change negative factors.

A POSITION FOR EACH PAIN

- **Poor circulation in the legs and pains during the night.** Sleep without a pillow and elevate the mattress at the feet (or foot of the bed) to improve blood flow to the legs.
- **Breathing problems.** To relieve breathing problems, the best position is to lie on your side, rather than on your back or belly.
- **Arthritis.** Those who suffer from arthritis should rest the affected area on a pillow or padded boxes.
- **Gastric reflex.** Avoid sleeping on your stomach. Avoid eating before going to bed. It's best to raise the upper part of the body while resting.

pillow, light and also extreme temperatures can contribute to sleepless nights.

■ **Excessive eating or drinking.** Eating foods high in saturated fats before going to bed, the use of alcohol or stimulants can contribute to unrestful sleep.

■ **Over-straining exercise or a sedentary lifestyle.** Exercising before going to bed can be a factor to insomnia. While at the same time not getting enough exercise can contribute to not getting a good night sleep.

■ **Bedtime habits.** Reading, listening to music, watching television or doing other stimulant activities while in bed can contribute to sleepless nights.

■ **Illness or medical problems.** It is not uncommon for people experiencing illness or medical problems to suffer from insomnia. Low sugar levels, thyroid problems, breathing problems, and some medications can cause or exacerbate insomnia.

REM SLEEP

During REM sleep we dream, this process can occur at any stage in the sleeping cycle. In REM, which lasts for short spurts of time, our breathing becomes more rapid, irregular, and shallow, our eyes jerk rapidly in various directions, and our limb muscles become temporarily paralyzed. During REM we relieve daily tensions, thus it is necessary to maintain a healthy mental state.

Changing your lifestyle

To treat insomnia, which can cause physical, mental and emotional problems, the first thing you must do is to adopt healthy habits and to create a positive environment for good sleep.

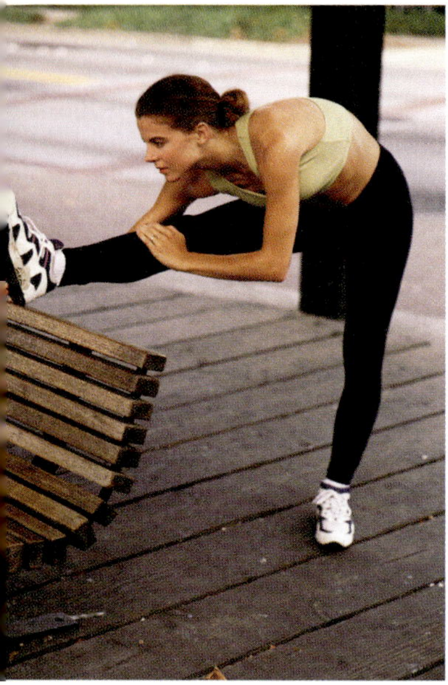

Changing daily habits doesn't happen over night. It's important to have a healthy outlook and consider the negative and positive results of your habits. This outlook will help you change habits and rest better.

To sleep better it's good to:

- Avoid drinking caffeinated or alcoholic beverages for several hours before bedtime. Although alcohol may initially act as a sedative, it can interrupt normal sleep patterns. The same for cigarettes. You may want to consider quitting all together. Smoking congests the respiratory airways and inflames their mucous lining, obstructing the flow of oxygen and contributing to insomnia.

- Do not overeat before going to bed, digestive process can disrupt the sleep cycle.
- Do not get out of bed when you have trouble sleeping. Do not eat or drink when you can't sleep. It's best to stay lying down, in a warm and dark room.
- Don't "catch up" on your sleep during the free days by sleeping more. Some

people use their weekend to sleep-in till noon. This kind of behaviour changes your internal biological clock.

- Don't go to bed when you have a lot on your mind. If you have a habit of making a to-do-list for the next day, make the list a few hours before going to bed, so you go to bed with a clear head.
- Make your bedroom primarily a place for sleeping. It is not a good idea to use your bed for paying bills, doing work, etc. Help your body recognize that this is a place for rest or intimacy.
- Don't get up earlier than you normally do. If you wake up before your normal time, you should try to go back to sleep, staying in a dark, warm room.
- Wake up when you are supposed to, although you might want to go back to sleep. It's not recommended to take a nap during the day.
- Organize your day so that you complete the most taxing activities during the morning or early afternoon, when you have more energy.

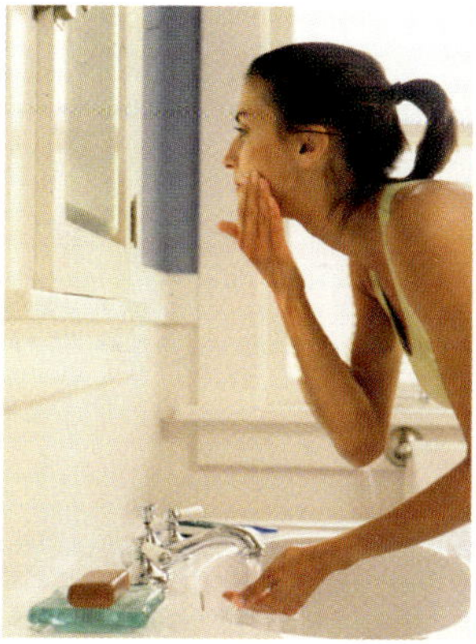

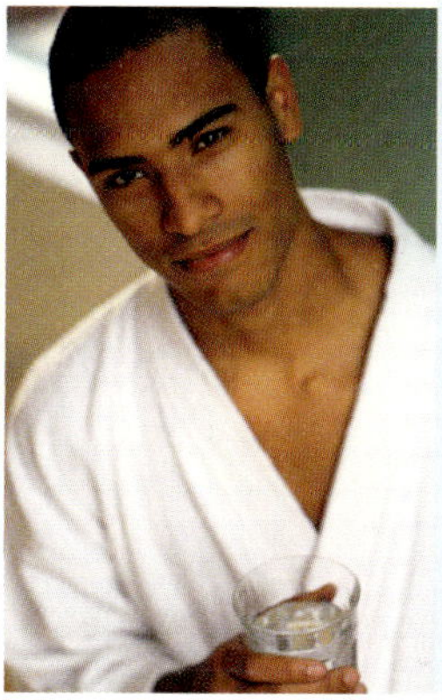

10 TIPS FOR A GOOD NIGHT'S SLEEP

1. Sleep in a comfortable position.
2. Avoid sleeping on your stomach.
3. Make sure your room is well ventilated and the temperature consistent.
4. Avoid noise and light.
5. Get a good pillow.
6. Do not use strong chemicals to clean in the bedroom.
7. Prohibit your dog or cat from sleeping in or on the bed.
8. Don't keep a lot of plants in the bedroom.
9. Never go to sleep without removing your makeup or perfume.
10. Avoid sleeping in recently painted rooms.

- Expose yourself to sunlight soon after waking up.
- Don't go to bed as soon as you feel tired. It's better to wait until your bedtime and don't alterate your sleep schedule.
- Set a regular and active routine, with physical activities and social events, so that your body gets tired from pleasant activities while keeping your head clear.
- Make sure to keep a regular schedule for meals, going to bed and waking up.
- Don't eat or drink when you should be sleeping, it can send contradictory signals to the biological rhythms.
- Exercise during the day, never close to bedtime. You should not exercise for four hours before going to bed.
- While you change your routine you should use the part of your day that you are least tired for work, physical and intellectual activities. It's healthy to divide your day into three parts: work, rest and sleep. Over time, your work-rest-sleep routine will normalize to help you be more productive.
- These tips will not create any side effects to your health.

INCORPORATE BEDTIME RITUALS

Taking a warm shower, a few minutes of reading, listening to soft music, lighting a candle or incense stick, drinking a cup of herbal tea or practicing relaxing techniques, cues your body that it's time to slow down and begin to prepare for sleep.

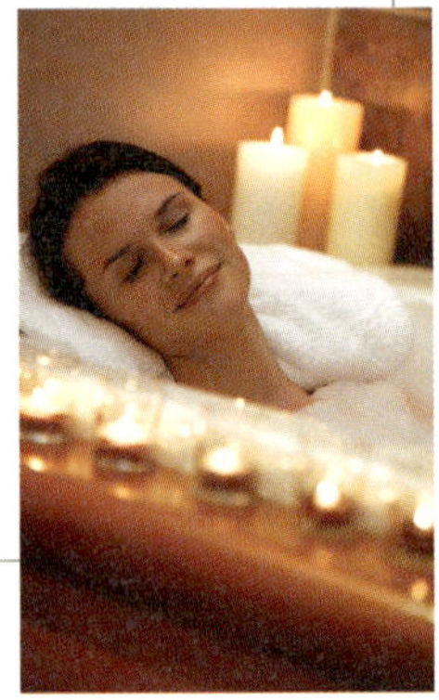

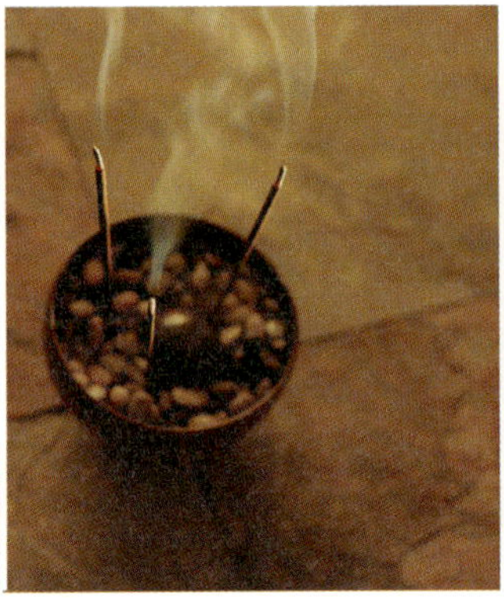

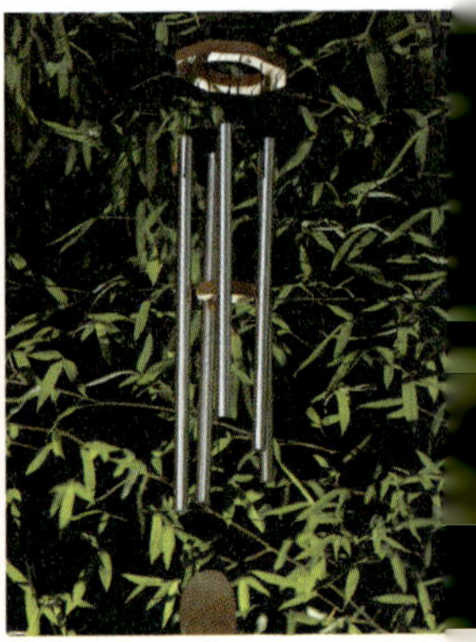

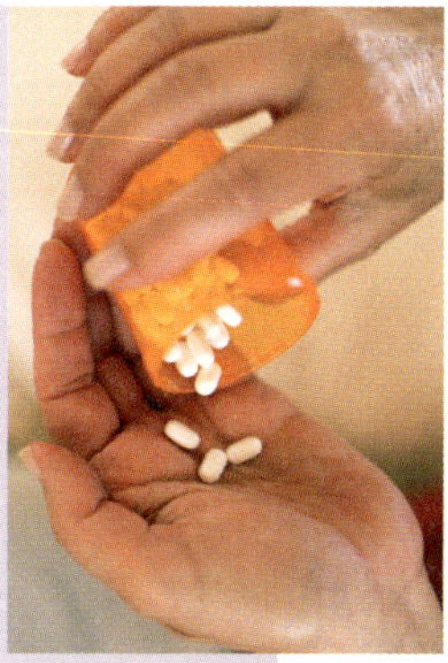

SLEEP AIDS

Avoid "over-the-counter" sleep aids, and make sure that your prescribed medications do not cause insomnia. There is little evidence that supplements and other over-the-counter "sleep aids" are effective. In some cases, there are safety concerns. Antihistamine sleep aids, in particular, have a long duration of action and can cause daytime drowsiness. Always talk to your doctor or healthcare practitioner about your concerns.

HOW LONG SHOULD I SLEEP?

Each person's sleep requirement is different. The average adult functions best with eight hours of sleep a night, but this varies with age and on an individual basis.

- Newborns can sleep up to 20 hours a day.
- Infants can sleep 16 hours a day.
- 6 year old children can sleep 12 hours a day.
- Adults can sleep 8 hours a day.
- Seniors generally don't need more than 6 hours sleep a day.

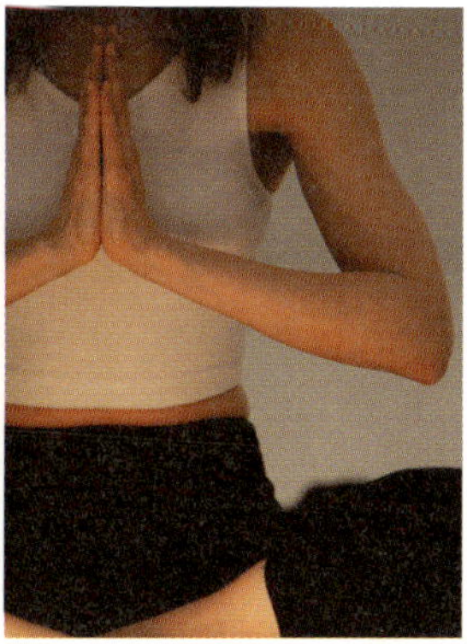

A GOOD SLEEPING POSITION

The best position is lying on your back, with your back straight. It's not recommended to sleep on your belly, this position can affect your back posture. Also, to breathe in this position you have to keep your neck twisted for several hours. Sleeping on your side (specially on your right side) can be an intermediary option to help you rest.

Visualizing to relax

Relaxing your body has the exact opposite physical effect of tension. When you enter a relaxing state, your heart beat slows, your breathing slows, your blood pressure lowers, your muscles relax and mental anxiety decreases.

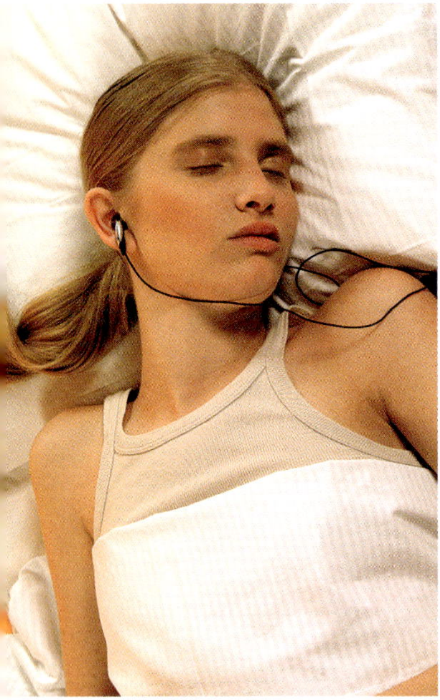

The first step for relaxing is to learn how to breathe in a correct manner, using your lungs to consciously keep a rhythm for breathing and connecting your breath to your emotions.
A simple and effective technique is abdominal breathing. By taking deep breaths the bottom of your lungs fills with air, moving your diaphragm downward and expanding your abdomen.

DREAMT RELAX

Visualization techniques to relax vary according to different schools and the people who use them. Here is a simple, effective technique:

1. Lie in bed, ready to sleep. Close your eyes and practice abdominal breathing (see *Relaxing breathing* box).

2. Concentrate and visualize your entire body, from the bottom to the top: toes, feet, legs, buttocks, stomach, back, chest, arms, shoulders, neck until you reach the face. When you exhale, release the tension in each part of your body and muscles.

3. Next, think about your breathing and whisper mindless things like "one", "peace" or phrases like "I am relaxed" or "I am calm", each time you exhale. It is also helpful to visualize a pleasant image while performing this technique.Thinking about repetitive or mindless things helps your brain to get distracted in order to fall asleep.

4. Each time a thought occurs, let it pass by like a cloud in the sky. Don't insist on your thoughts. Continue until you fall asleep.

RELAXING BREATHING

To practice proper abdominal breathing, begin by placing one of your hands on your chest and the other on your abdomen. Breath through your nose as indicated in the steps below. The hand on your abdomen will rise as your abdomen expands and your hand on your chest should remain immobile. Exhale through your mouth, with a whispering breath. To guide you better follow these steps:

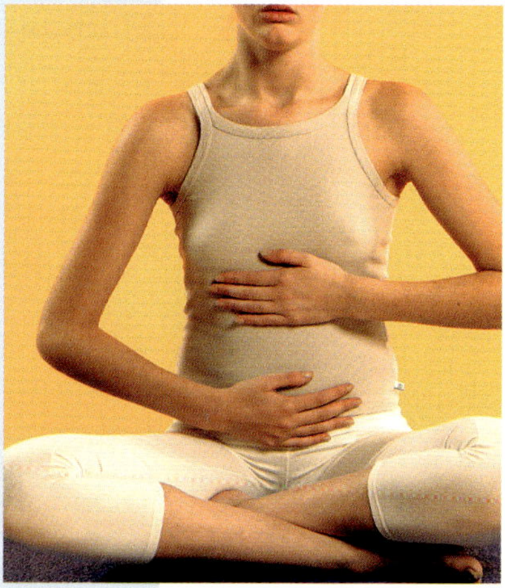

1. Take a deep breath through the nose expanding your abdomen.

2. Keep your breath in for a few seconds and slowly exhale, releasing the air in double the time you took to inhale.

You can also practice this exercise when lying down, with a book placed on your abdomen. You will see the book rises as air expands your abdomen and then slowly descends as you exhale.

Meditating for a good night sleep

Creative visualization and meditation are very efficient in fighting insomnia. Those who practice meditation say that, as time goes by, the sleep they get is deeper and more refreshing. They feel more alert and relaxed throughout the day.

✚ Using your imagination, visualization helps to create subjective realities (or images) relaxing your mind as a positive method to help you sleep more deeply and to improve your overall health. The following exercise is to help you relax and rest.

THE IDEAL PLACE

The objective of visualization is to create an imaginary place for your mind to take a "mental vacation". This can be for example, imagining a familiar landscape and add certain details (a hammock, music, palm trees) or a completely imaginary place. Once you've been able to create your mental vacation site, practice the following exercise. When you've completed the exercise, your imaginary place will have become even more detailed and will stay etched in your memory to use whenever you need it.

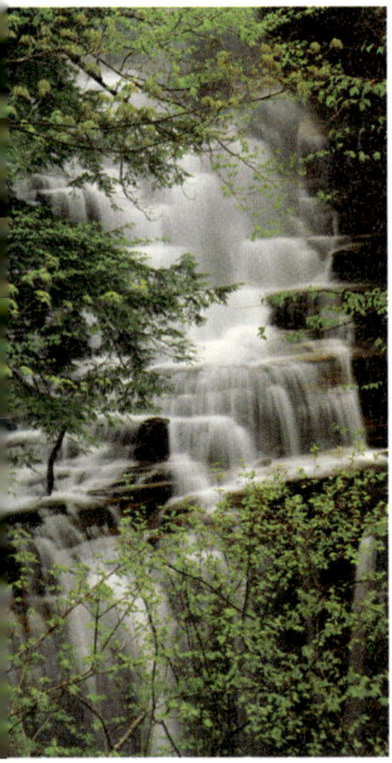

CLOSE YOUR EYES

Visualize number 3, three times:
Three… three… three… Your body has already relaxed.
Visualize number 2, three times:
Two… two… two…

Your mind is already relaxed.
Visualize number **1**, three times:
One… one… one…
When you've reached the first 1, you are learning to reach any mental image you wish.
Now go to your ideal place for rest.
Count from five to one. Once you count down you will enter a deeper, healthier relaxation.
Five… Four… Deeper and deeper
Three… Even deeper Two… One.

Every time you breath you feel the harmony and beauty of this place fill your lungs, bringing you a sense of pleasure, relaxation and peace. You feel as if your body is riding on waves of well-being. Each time you decide to go to this relaxing place, your body will relax with each breath.
When you feel you've reached a state of total tranquility, leave this place counting to five.
One…
Two…
Three…
Four…
Five.

When you reach five your body and mind will feel healthy and relaxed.
Record someone reading and repeating the steps, using a pleasant and slow voice to soothe and relax you. Listening to the phrases each night will help you follow the steps and bring on sleep.

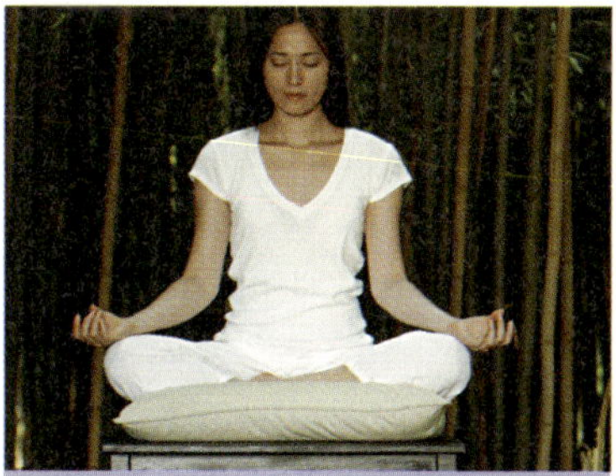

MEDITATION

Meditation is a technique to calm and relax your mind, direct your concentration to a healing element away from worries. When beginning meditation, a practitioner or guide is needed. Meditation is recommended for sleeping disorders.
Some health benefits of meditation:

- Decreases anxiety and stress.
- Helps you explore your inner emotions and physical state.
- Deepens the realm of the spiritual, bringing a state of harmony and union between the mind, body and spirit.

Improving your rest with yoga

Yoga is a technique dating back thousands of years. Its philosophical principles are based on creating harmony between the mind, body and spirit. Regularly practicing yoga can improve your health, help you relax better and can treat insomnia.

Hatha yoga, the path of physical yoga, is the most popular branch of yoga in the West. It uses physical poses or *asanas*, breathing techniques or *pranayamas*, energy flows *bandas* and psychic gestures *mudras*. Each yoga pose is thought to improve your body's functions while at the same time increasing your clarity and mental concentration. The poses also prepare the body and mind for meditation, a state that helps bring on sleep.

The Bridge

It may help to stretch the spinal column and relieve tension where we most often store it in the back.

1. *In a lying position, with your arms extended next to your body and your knees bent, feet together, keeping the balls of your feet pressed against the floor and as close to the buttocks as possible.*

2. *Tighten your buttocks and inhale while keeping your feet pressed to the floor; exhale while you lift up your hips, keeping your knees pressed together and lifting your belly button as high as you can. Stay in this position inhaling and exhaling three times, each time you inhale try to lift your belly button higher. Exhale and lower your body.*

1

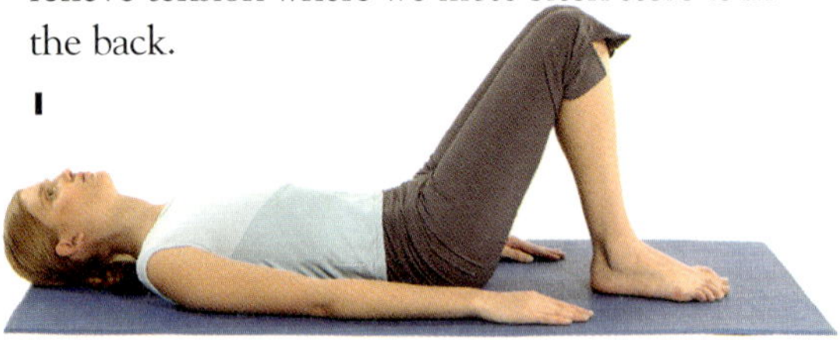

2

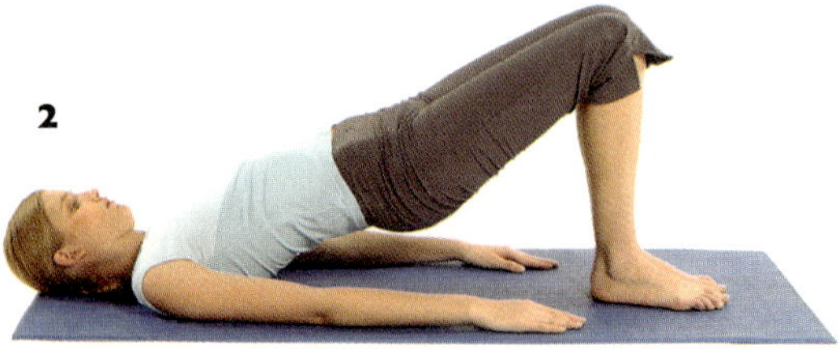

Another way to do this position is to take your ankles in your hands and while you inhale raise your buttocks and trunk; lower your buttocks when you exhale. Repeat three times.

The Plow

This pose may help to relax, calm you and facilitate digestion, making it a good *asana* to help you sleep. In addition it nourishes the spinal nerves and gives flexibility to the spine, neck and back, helping you to sleep better.

1. *Begin the position lying on your back, with your legs together, arms down by your sides next to your body and the palms of your hands pressed to the floor. Bring your chin toward your chest and press your back muscles to the floor. Inhale through your nose and raise your legs up until they are at a 90 degree angle with your torso. Exhale, then inhale and bring your hips off the floor, supporting your back with your hands.*

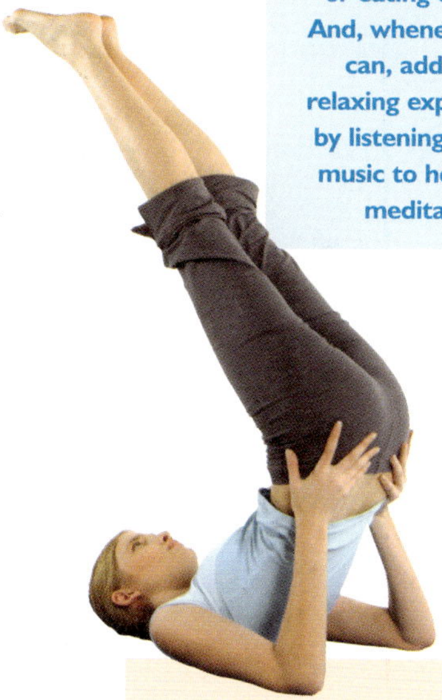

2. *Without bending your knees, stretch out your legs by bringing them behind your head, until your toes touch the floor. Your arms should stay forward, with the palms of your hands pressed to the floor. Stay in this position breathing slowly and deeply. Next, inhale through your nose and slowly lower your legs while you exhale. Concentrate on how each segment of your backbone presses against the floor.*

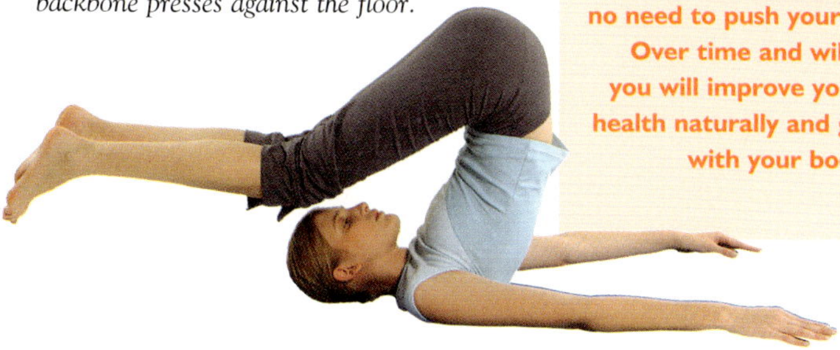

GETTING READY

For these exercises to completely relax you and to bring on sleep, it's best to do them two hours before going to bed or eating dinner. And, whenever you can, add to a relaxing experience by listening to soft music to help you meditate.

GENTLE EXERCISE

Yoga is a discipline designed to improve your flexibility and harmony. The exercises use gentle movements without straining your body. When practicing the *asanas* remember not to strain yourself. There is no need to push yourself too far. Over time and willpower, you will improve your body's health naturally and get in tune with your body.

Rocking chair

This yoga exercise is always done at the beginning of a yoga session, before beginning other *asanas*, to stretch out the body. It is also indicated for practicing a few hours before going to bed because it promotes relaxation and resting well.

1. Begin sitting on the floor (or on a padded mat); bend your legs, leave the soles of your feet pressed against the floor. Wrap your hands around the part of your leg behind the knee, leaving your thumbs outward. Keep your chin pressed to your chest to avoid back problems. Slowly lean back to give you momentum.

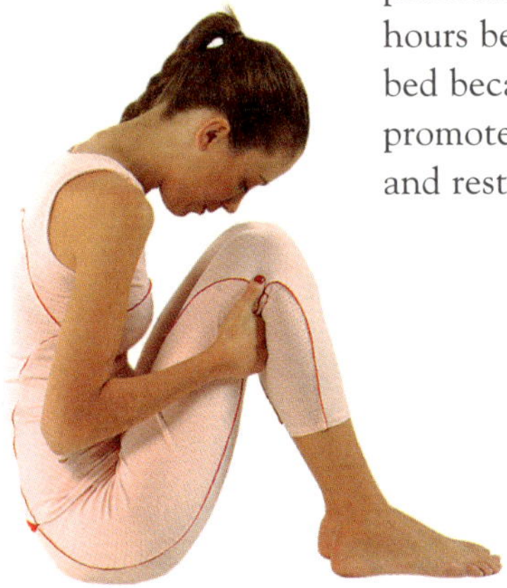

2. Next, push your legs back with your hands, gently inhaling, the body goes back until your back is off the mat, with your legs still bent and your chin pressed to your chest. Next, exhale and return to the initial position.
You may like to practice this pose 10 or 15 times.

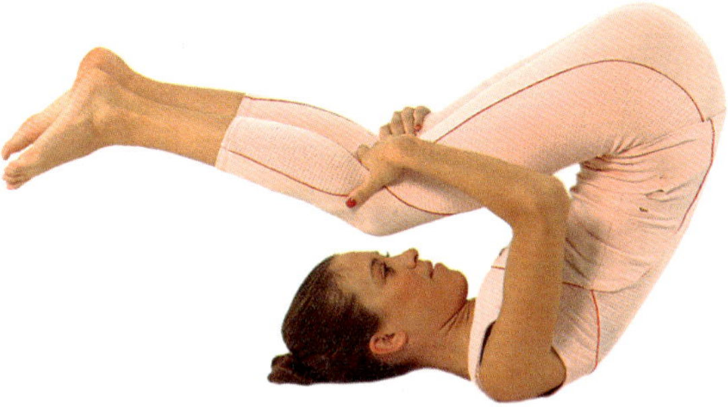

In the future, when you are more familiar with the movement, you will be able to take your legs all the way back until the tips of your toes touch the floor behind your head. Return while you exhale, never lifting the chin from the chest. You may like to repeat this position 15 times, always keeping your chin pressed to your chest, inhaling as you go back and expelling your breath as you go forward. Afterward, lie down on the mat and relax.

THE CHILD'S POSE

This *asana* relaxes the entire body and brings a sense of total well-being, while at the same time relieving stomach pain and helping to bring on sleep.

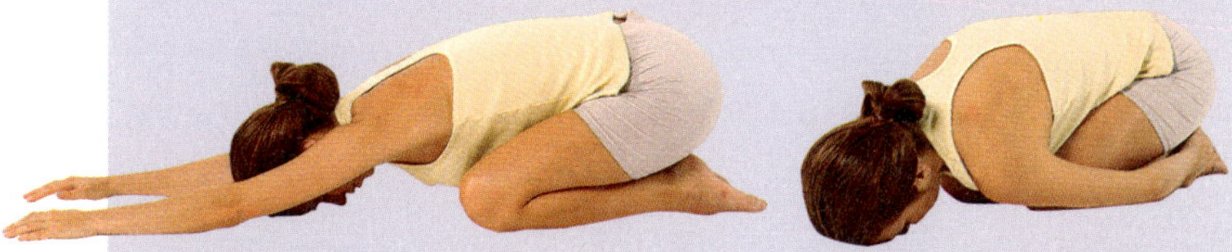

***1.** Kneel down and sit on your feet with your heels pointing outward. Your knees should be separated, about the width of your hips. Inhale as you lift your arms above your head and exhale while you bring your torso down to your thighs. Place your forehead, palms of your hands and forearms on the floor, while keeping your shoulders relaxed.*

***2.** Next, bring your arms behind and keep them relaxed next to the body. Stay in this position for however long you like, breathing softly and keeping your mind on your spinal column.*

The Tree

This position may help concentration, bringing confidence and elasticity to the body. It also works with the body's balance, mental stability and spiritual harmony. It is practiced with your back straight and constantly looking forward. Always concentrate on your breathing and use very slow and controlled movements. Little by little you will gain confidence.

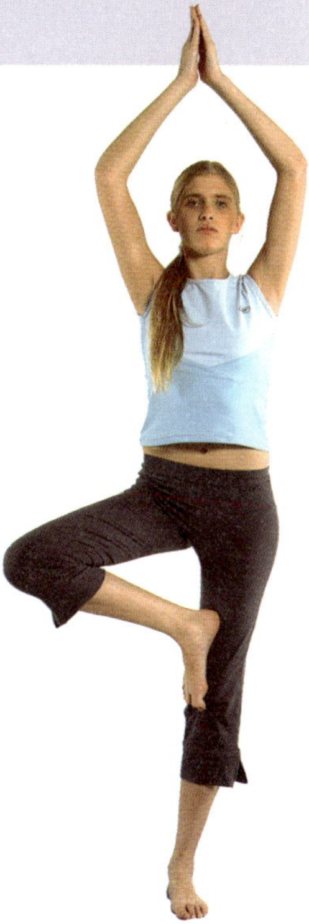

Stand with your legs apart, putting all of your weight on your left foot. Place your right foot on the inside of your left thigh. Once you have balance, bring your hands together toward your chest, breathing slowly; while you inhale lift up your hands –always with your palms together– above your head. Stay in this position as long as you can. Next, return to the initial position by doing the steps backward. Repeat the position, but with your other leg.

Do-in and... get ready to relax!

Do-in is a combination of techniques based on *shiatsu*, called the "physiotherapy of contact". The technique can revitalize and relieve physical and mental tensions.

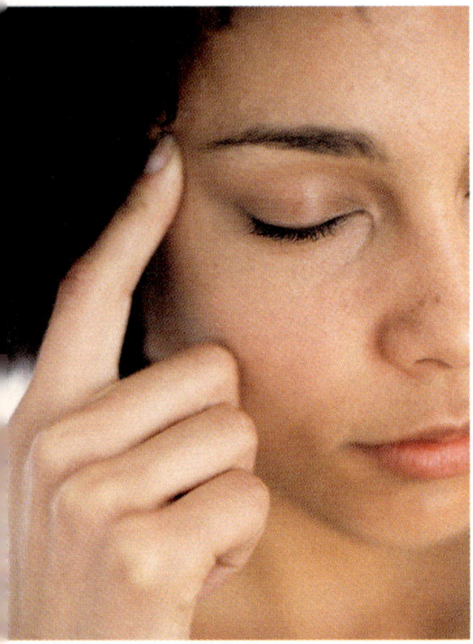

Shiatsu means "finger pressure" in Japanese. Using the rhythmic pressing of acupressure points for short periods, this *shiatsu* technique is a treatment which works on the meridians of the body to put our *chi* or life energy in balance. This treatment regulates imbalances in the *chi* that can provoke illnesses. *Shiatsu*, through *do-in* massages can correct internal imbalances, especially those that are produced by the tensions and stress that in many cases cause insomnia. Practicing the following exercises before going to bed can induce a deep relaxing state making a harmonious night's sleep possible.

TO RELAX YOUR NECK

In a sitting position on the floor, with your legs crossed, back straight and your eyes closed, imagine that the point of your nose is a pencil. Use your nose to draw big circles, with slow movements, going from the right to the left. After tracing various circles, rest your head looking toward the front and then continue to the right.

This exercise not only relaxes your neck and brings well-being but it also releases tight, achy muscles that can keep you from sleeping.

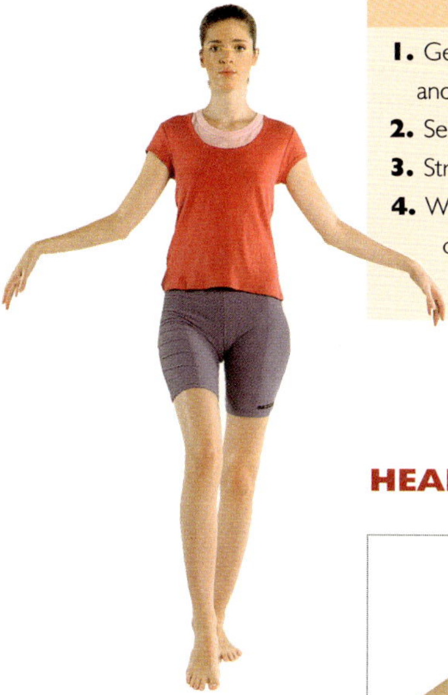

TO BEGIN

1. Gently pat the body, patting the arms, hands, legs and feet.
2. Separate your legs and relax your knees.
3. Straighten the back and relax your shoulders.
4. With your eyes closed, breath naturally and concentrate on how your body feels, paying special attention to the areas that are tense and achy.

HEAD AND FACE

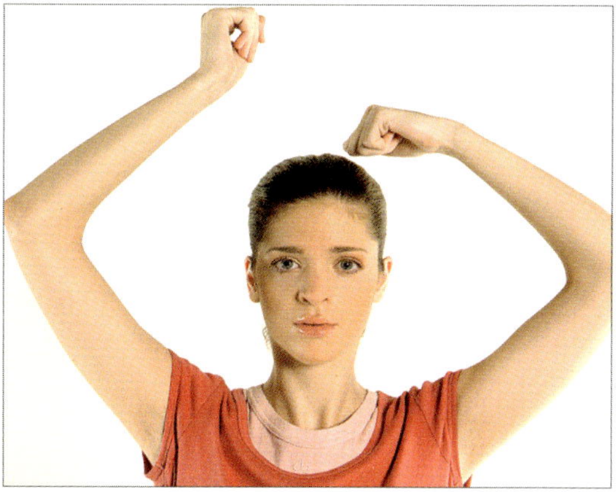

1. With your fists partly closed, relax your wrists and gently tap on the crown of your head.

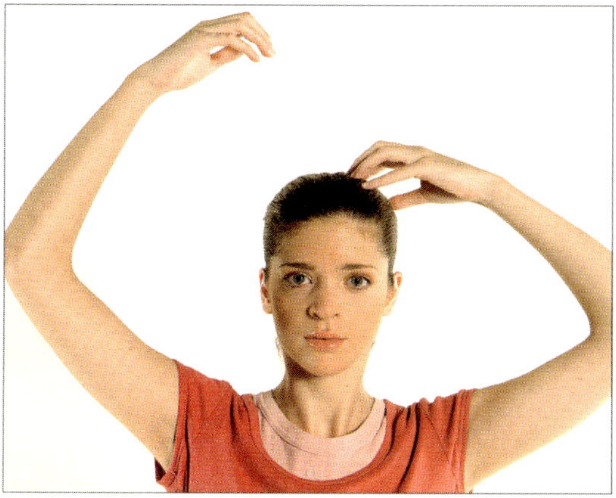

2. Next, continue tapping gently on your head with your hands open, using your fingertips or the palms of your hands. Cover your entire head with taps, including the temples, forehead and neck.

3. *To stimulate the meridians that cross your head, run your fingers through your hair several times.*

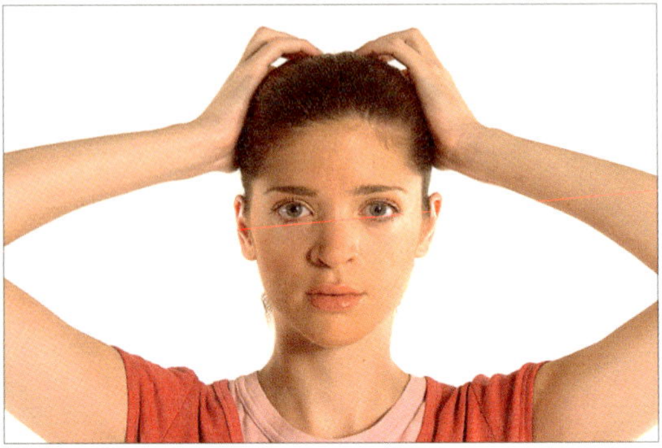

4. *Continue on your forehead, pressing with your fingertips, moving from the center of your forehead to your temples. Repeat three times.*

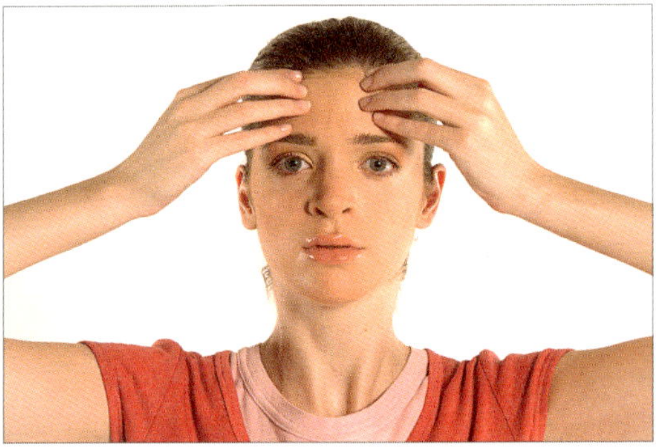

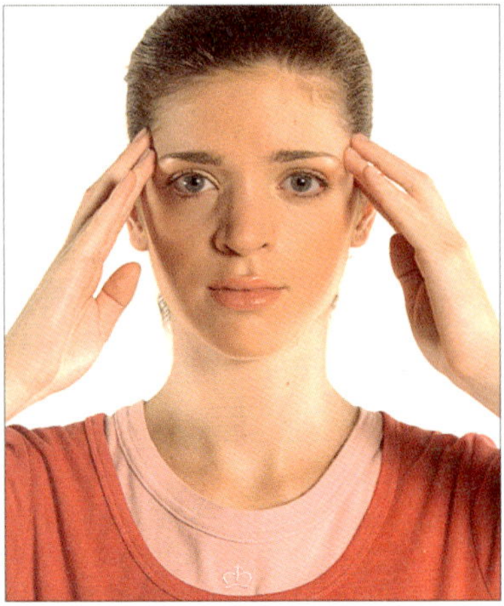

5. *Gently and repeatedly massage your temples. Make sure to relax your eyebrows and shoulders.*

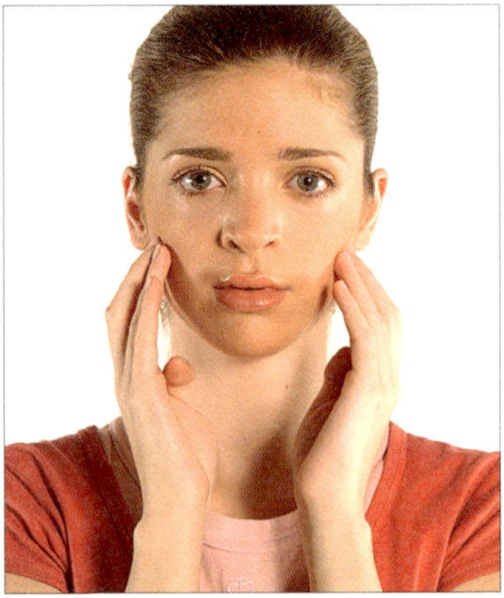

6. *Now massage your cheeks, moving from your temples to your jaw.*

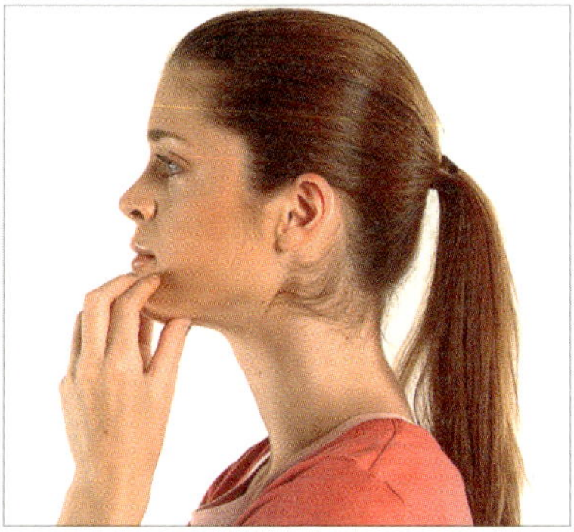

7. *Apply pressure on your jaw, from the center to the sides, relaxing and stimulating your saliva glands.*

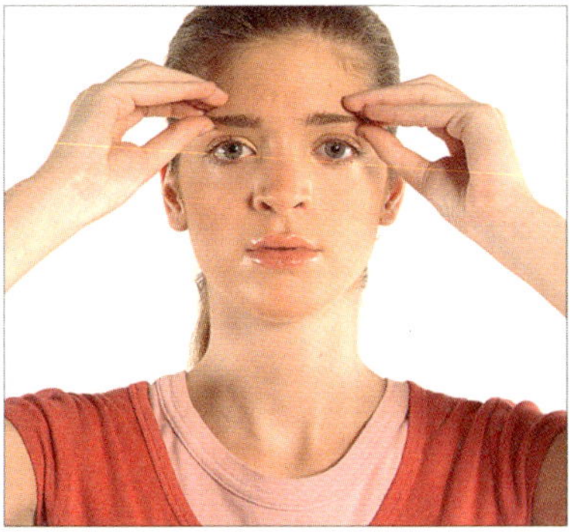

8. *Apply pressure with your index fingers and thumbs of both hands on your eyebrows, from the center moving outward. Repeat several times.*

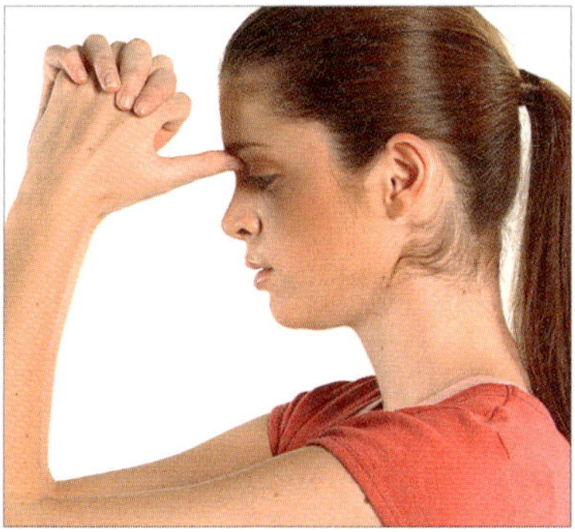

9. *Apply pressure on the point between your eyebrows with your thumbs.*

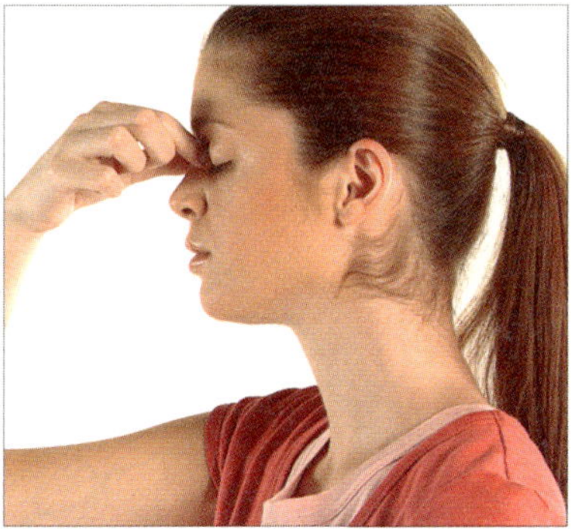

10. *With your index finger and thumb, pinch the bridge of your nose and the outset of your eyes. This exercise is ideal when your vision is exhausted.*

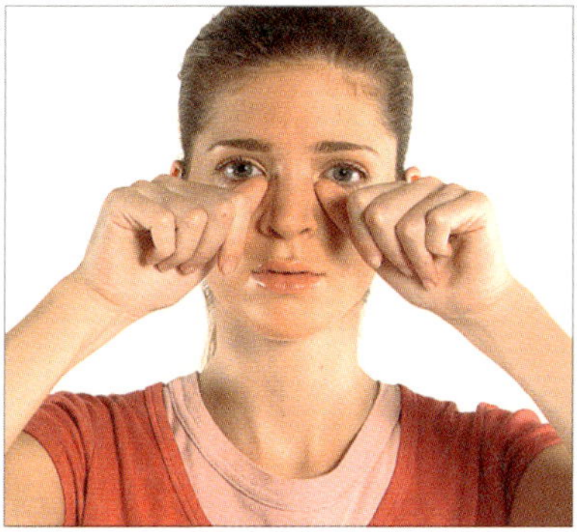

11. *To clear a congested nose, press your thumbs against your nose, keeping your other fingers bent. Inhale while you quickly rub your thumbs downward. Repeat three times.*

NECK

1. *Place the palm of your hand on your neck and apply firm, circular massages.*

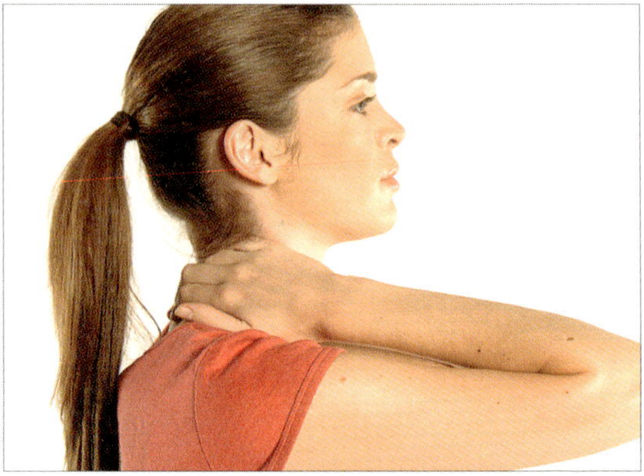

2. *With your thumbs, apply pressure on the base of the skull. Move the pressure upward.*

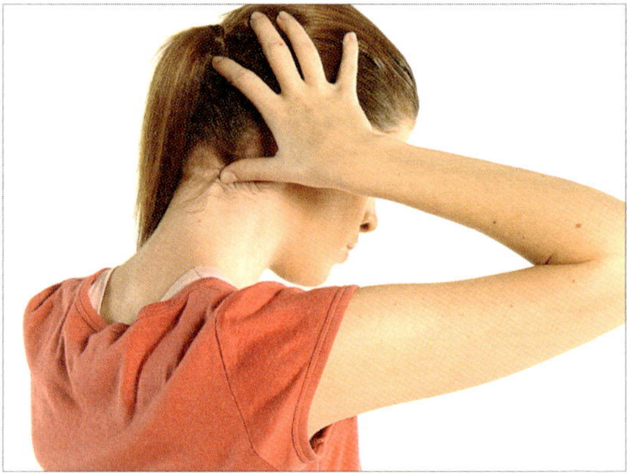

3. *Rub your fingers over your muscle fibers at the base of your skull to loosen the muscles and tendons in the area.*

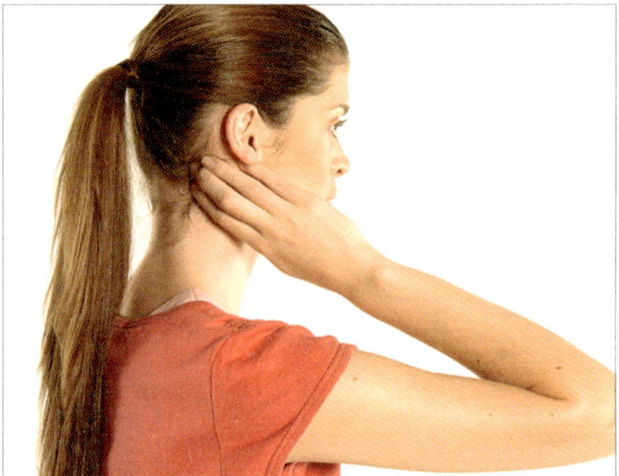

SHOULDERS, ARMS AND HANDS

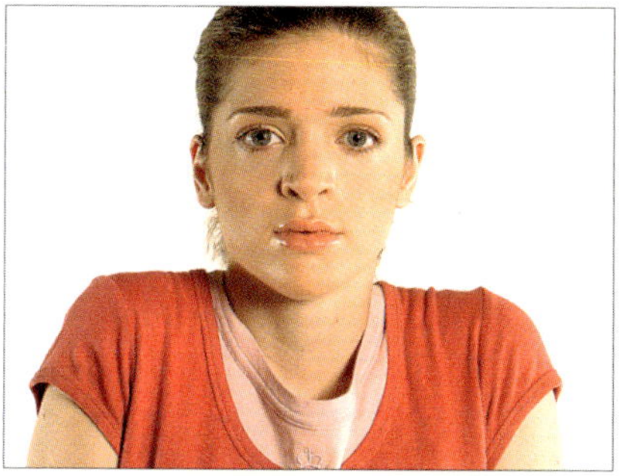

1. First, shake the arms outward to relax them. Next, lift your shoulders, inhaling. While you exhale completely relax your shoulders as you drop them back down. Repeat three times.

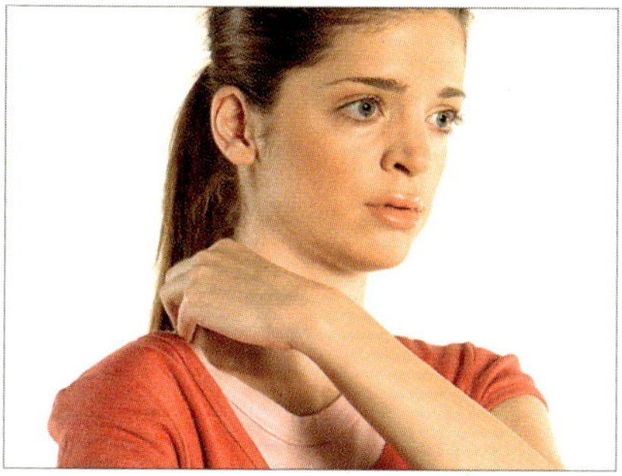

2. Support your left elbow with your right hand. With your left hand, gently hit your right shoulder, with a lose fist.

3. With your middle finger apply pressure to the highest point on your shoulder. **Warning.** *This self-massage is not recommended during pregnancy.*

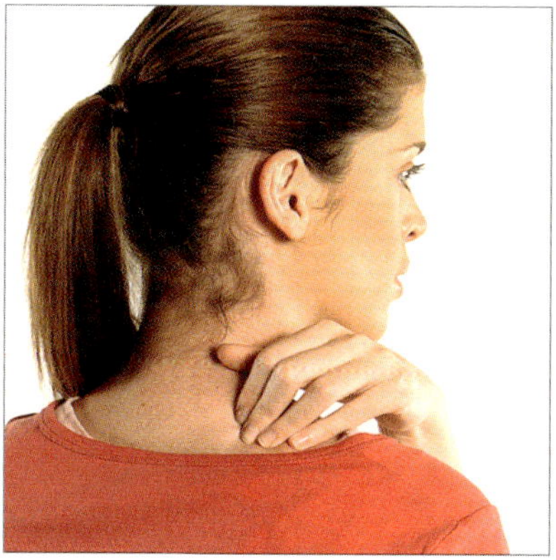

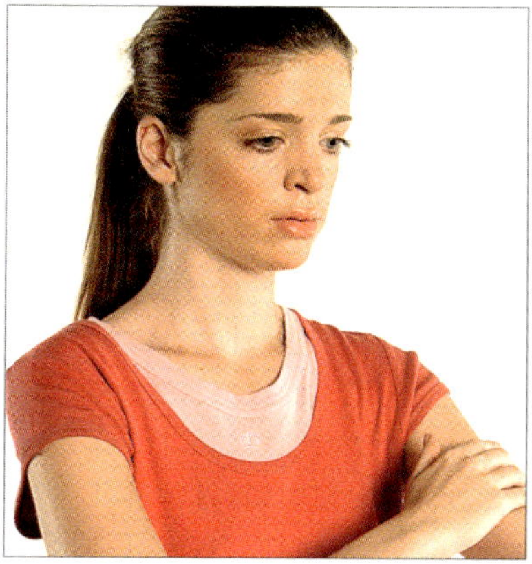

4. With your arms stretched out, apply gentle taps with the palm of your hand on the inside of each of your arms, moving from your shoulder all the way down to the palm of your hand. Repeat on both arms.

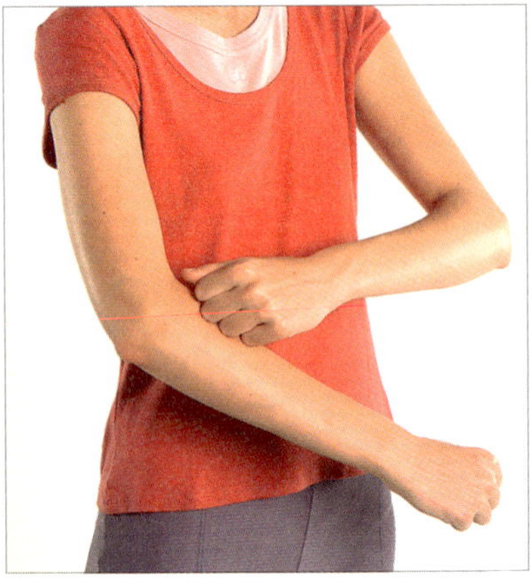

5. *Turn your arm over and hit your outer arm, moving up from the hand to the shoulder.*

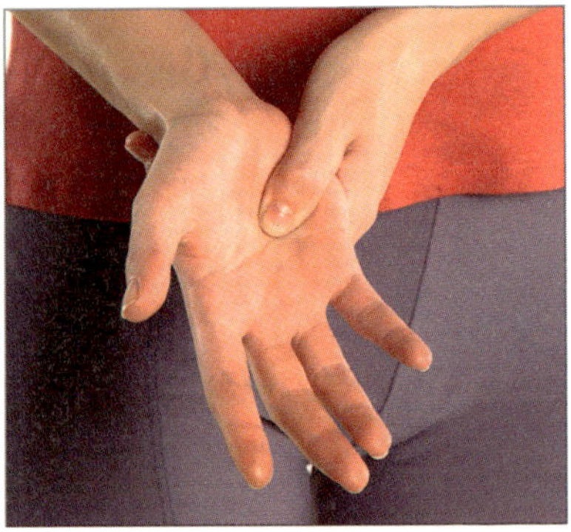

6. *With your left thumb, massage the palm of your right hand (you tend to store a lot of tension in this point). Next, repeat on the other hand.*

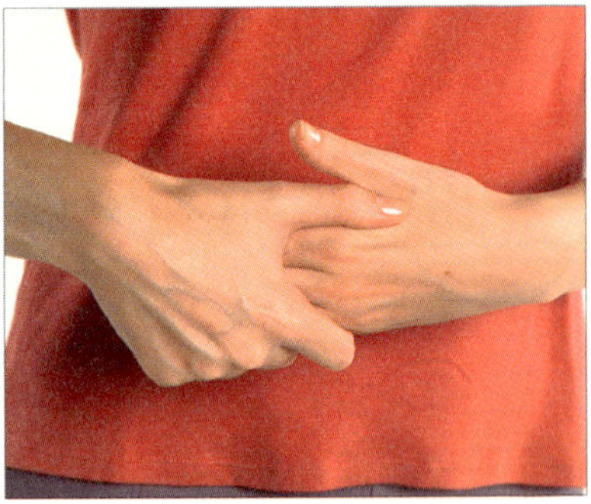

7. *On each hand, apply pressure to the point between the index finger and the thumb. This can cause a sense of general well-being and fights stress and diarrhea.* ***Warning.*** *It is not advised to use this massage during pregnancy.*

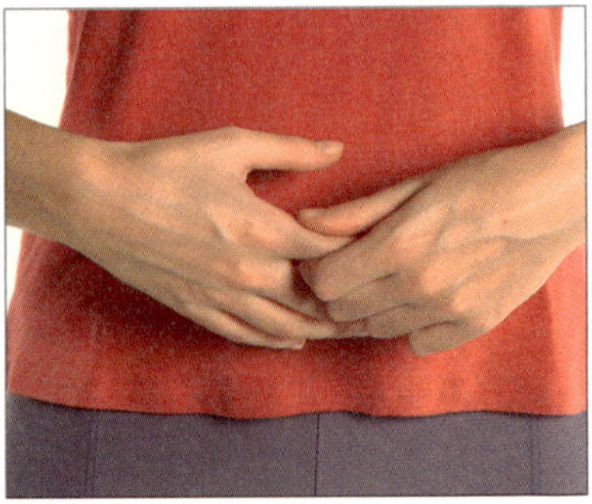

8. *With your index finger and thumb, apply pressure and gently massage the joints of each of your fingers.*

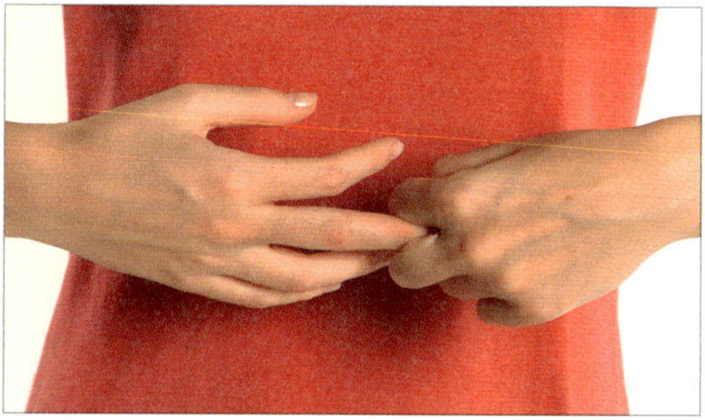

9. Stretch each finger of both hands. This exercise fights stress and tension.

CHEST, ABDOMEN, AND BACK

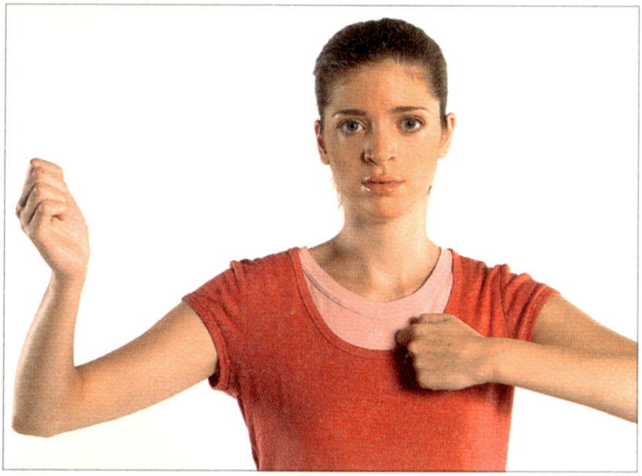

1. Straighten your back and push out your chest. Gently tap on the chest, on and around the breasts or chest muscles and along the ribcage.

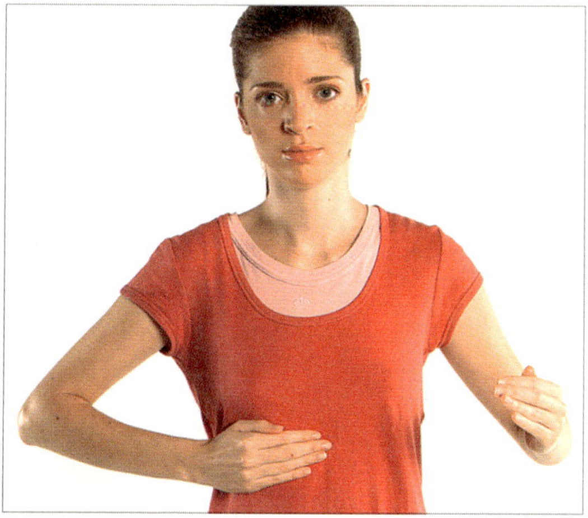

2. After taking in a deep breath, repeat the previous exercise, this time giving out an "ah" sound as you exhale.

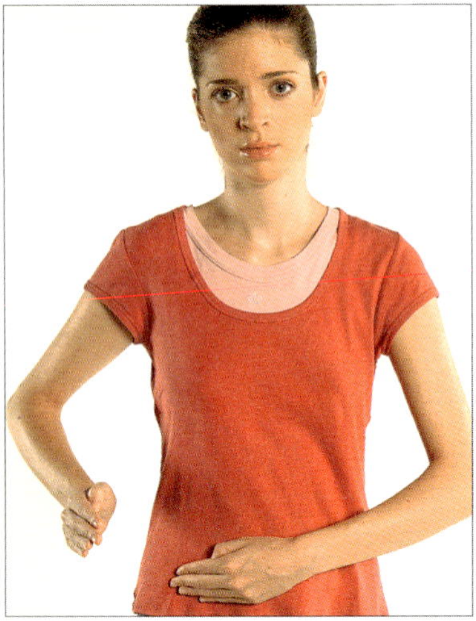

3. *Continue tapping downward until you reach the abdomen, in clock-wise movements, moving down on the left side and upward on the right side. This will accompany the flow of circulation and digestion.*

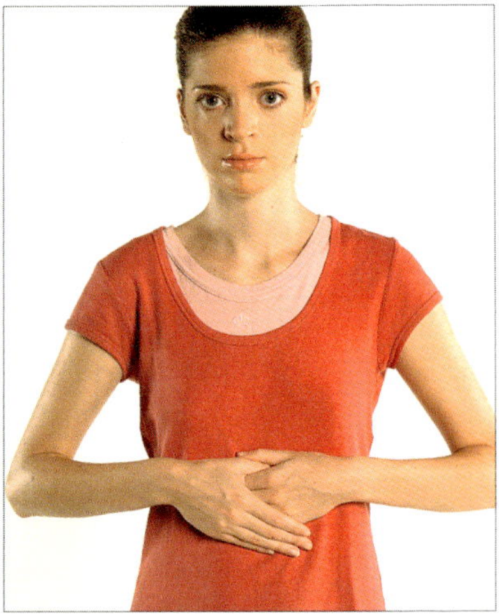

4. *Place one hand on the other and gently massage the abdomen.*

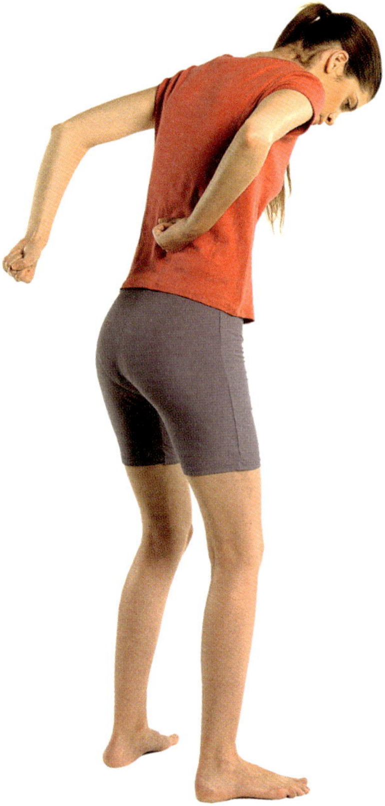

5. *Place your hands on the back, below the thorax, where your kidneys are located. Rub several times, until you feel heat from your hands on your body. Next, apply small taps with a relaxed fist.*

6. *Bend forward, and place your hand on one of your knees. With the back of your other hand lightly tap on the lumbar region between the ribs and the base of the spinal column. This is a therapy to clear your mind and activate brain signals that stimulate the nervous system.*

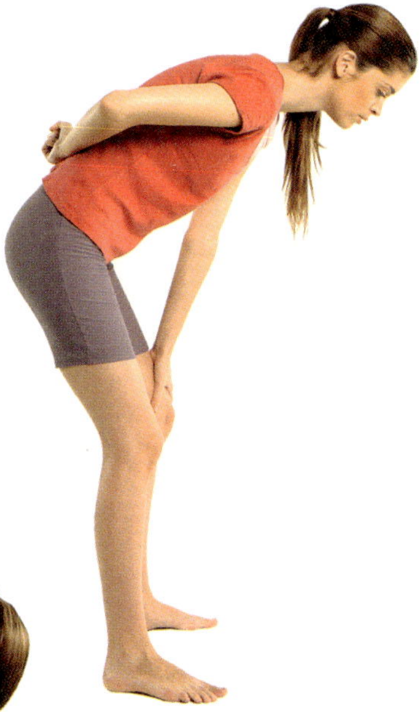

LEGS

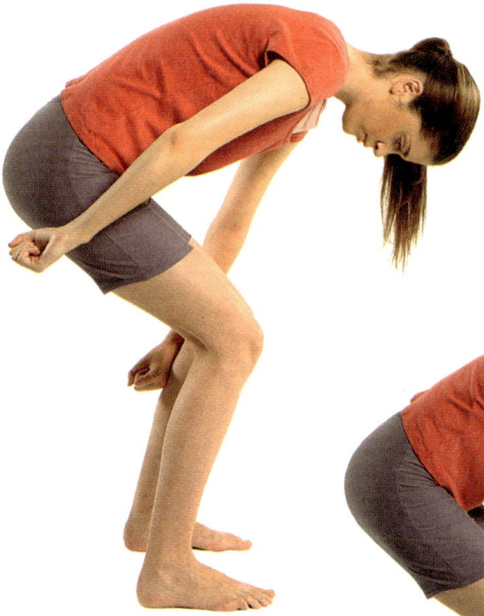

1. *With a loose fist, apply gentle blows along the backs of the legs from the hips to the calves.*

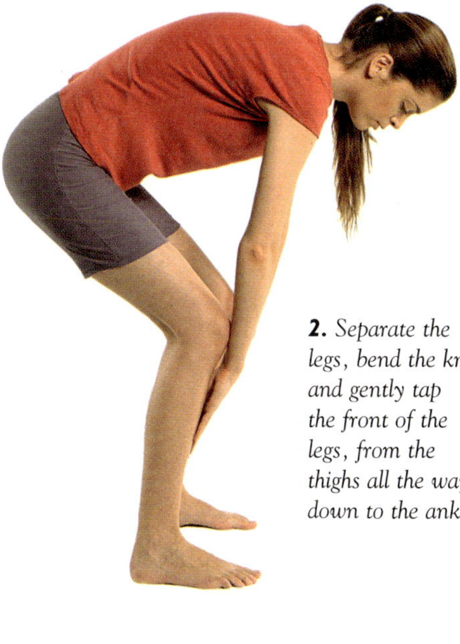

2. *Separate the legs, bend the knees and gently tap the front of the legs, from the thighs all the way down to the ankles.*

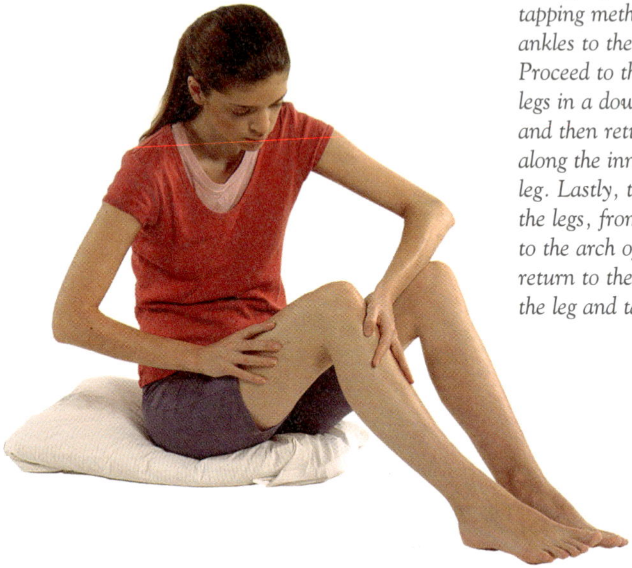

3. *Now on the inner part of the legs, gently use the same tapping method from the ankles to the groin. Proceed to the outside of the legs in a downward direction and then return upward along the inner part of the leg. Lastly, tap the front of the legs, from the thigh down to the arch of the foot, then return to the inner part of the leg and tap upward.*

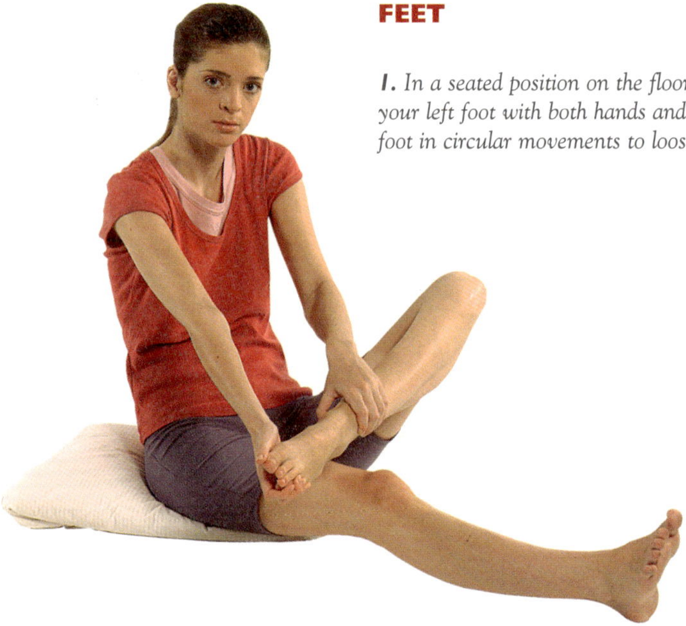

FEET

1. *In a seated position on the floor, hold onto your left foot with both hands and move the foot in circular movements to loosen the joints.*

2. *Next, with your thumbs massage the base of your foot. Apply special pressure on the point a third of the distance from the base of the second toe and the edge of the ball of the foot.*

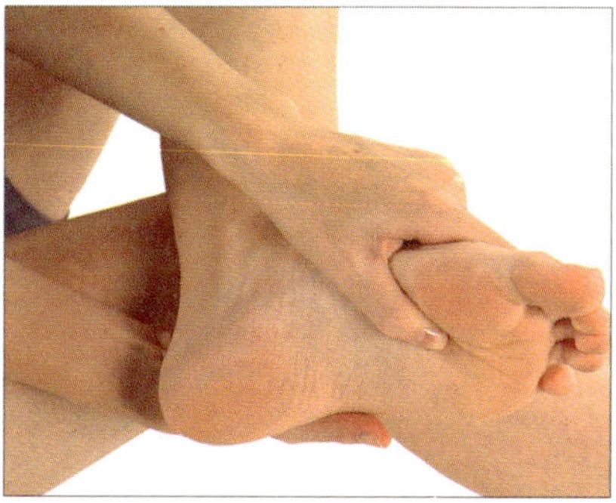

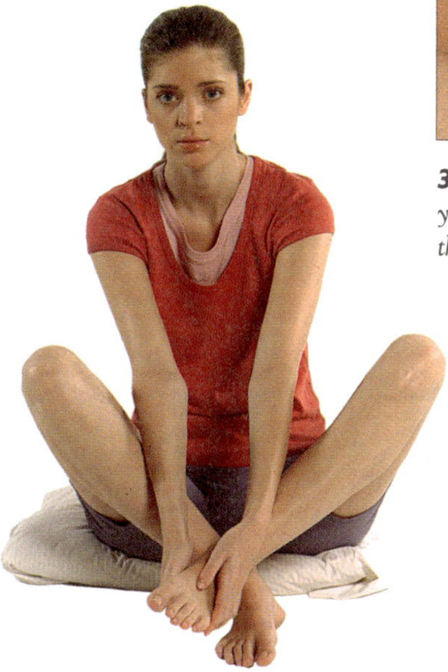

3. *Press on the point between your big toe and second toe on the front of the foot.*

TO FINISH A SESSION

As when you started, stand up and gently shake out your body. Standing with your legs spread shoulders width apart and your knees slightly bent, straighten your back to facilitate the flow of the *chi*. Allow your mind to travel throughout your body and feel your relaxed state.

4. *Wrap your hands around your left foot and rub it. Continue using the same technique on the right foot.*

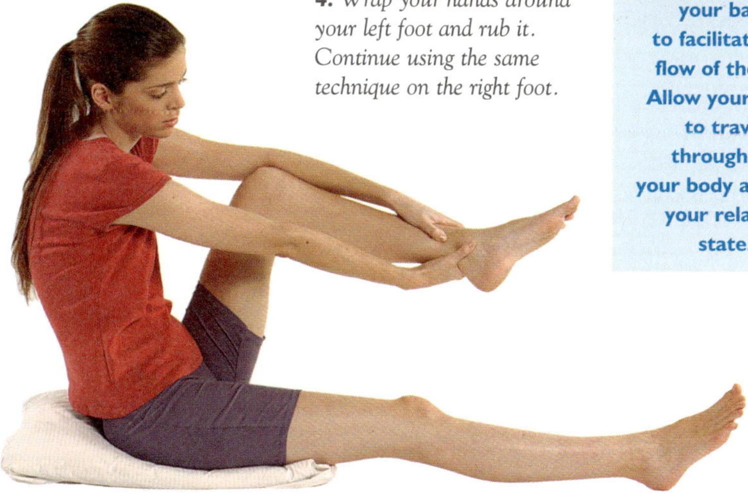

Reflexes and well-being

This natural healing art is based on the principles and study of the belief that there are reflexes in the body –especially on the feet– that correspond to the body's organs and glands. Applying stimulation and pressure to the feet, can affect the health of other parts of the body. The following are exercises that help to fight insomnia.

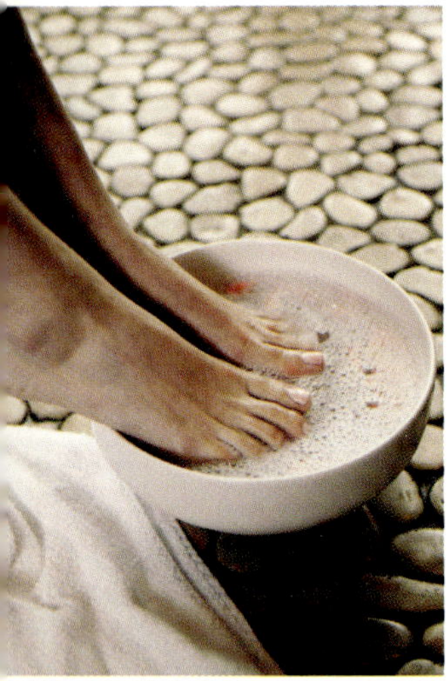

After washing your feet begin by massaging them –first one foot and then the other– from the base of your foot all the way to your ankle. Take one of your feet in your hand and roll your foot to get rid of tension. Continue by massaging each one of your toes, one by one and then massage the base of your foot.

SIDE EFFECTS

You shouldn't use these massage techniques if you suffer from:

- *Fevers or serious diseases.*
- *Blood clotting or lymphatic and vascular inflammations.*
- *Gangrene in the hands or feet.*
- *Athletes foot or foot fungus.*
- *Pregnancy with risk of miscarriage.*

To fight anxiety, to relax you and induce sleep. Wrap each foot with both hands and press with your thumbs on the point that corresponds to your solar plexus that is located in the center of your foot. This exercise can be done as a self-massage or by another person.

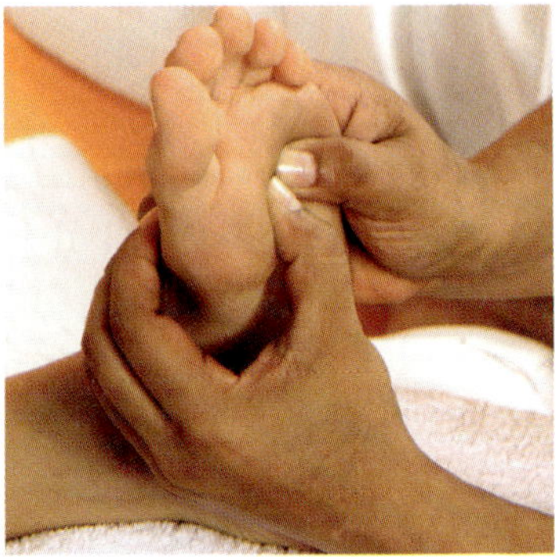

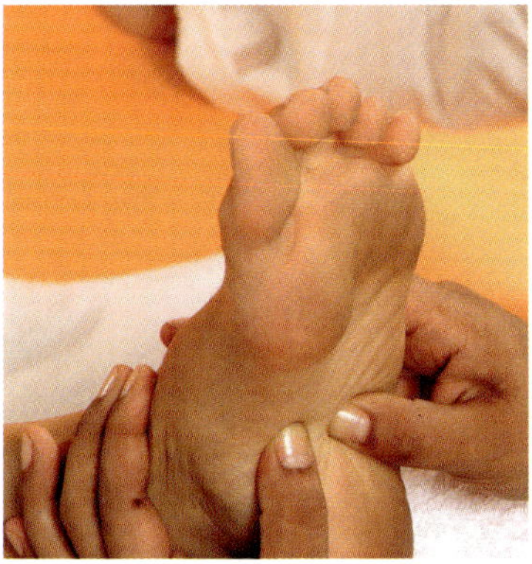

For insomnia and digestive problems. Wrap your hands around the foot and with your thumbs, press on the points that correspond to the stomach, which are located in the center of the foot (see diagram).

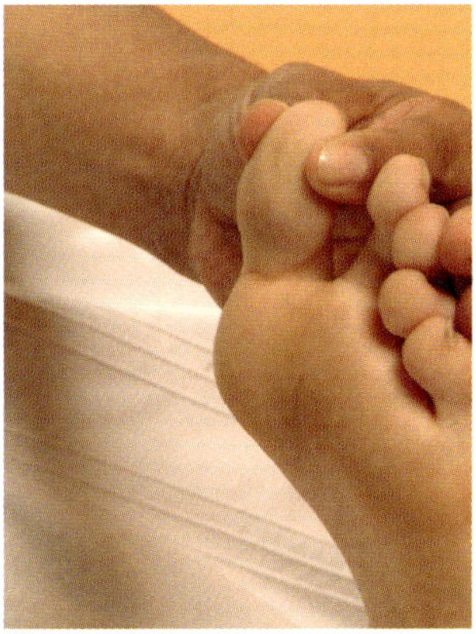

To relieve worries and improve mental clarity to help bring on sleep. Press with the thumb and the index finger on edges of the big toe on each foot, at the points of the foot that correspond to the head.

FOOT REFLEXOLOGY

For reflexology to be used as a therapy to help you sleep, you should first massage the entire foot and the areas that relax the body. Next, pay special attention to the points that correspond to the solar plexus and diaphragm to release anxiety. Massage the edges of the big toes, points that correspond to the head area and contribute to the energetic balance that helps to bring on sleep.

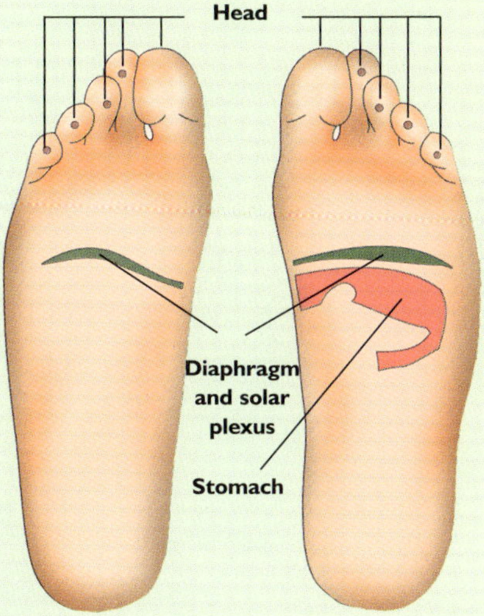

Restful massages

These massages can be used as a powerful tool to help your body to rest up and to repair itself.

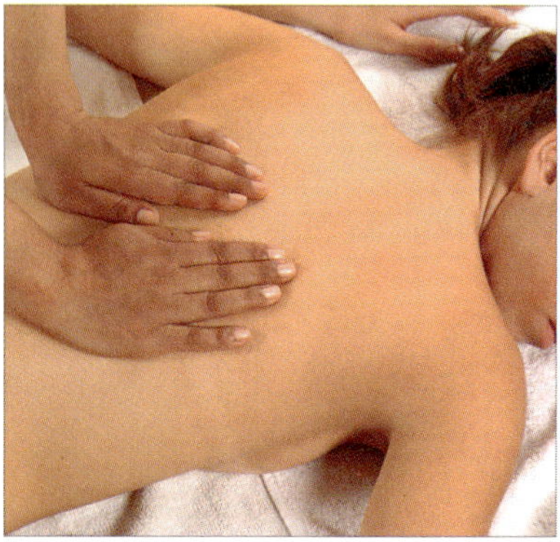

1. First pass your hands over the entire back, to detect tension.

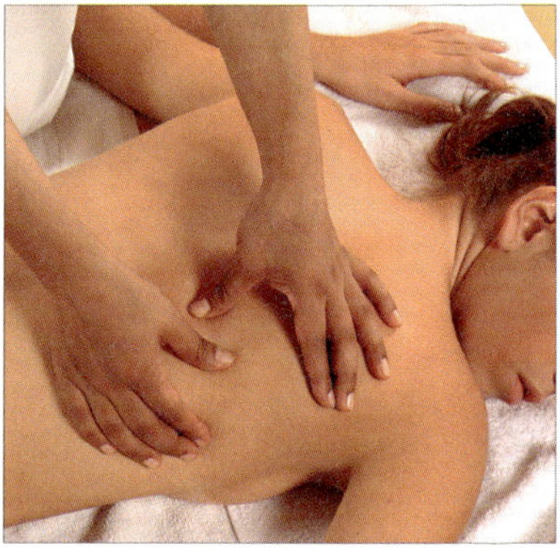

2. Where you feel knots, massage with the tips of your thumbs, using repetitive motions (like kneading with your thumbs). Next, use circular, clock-wise motions, to get rid of tension.

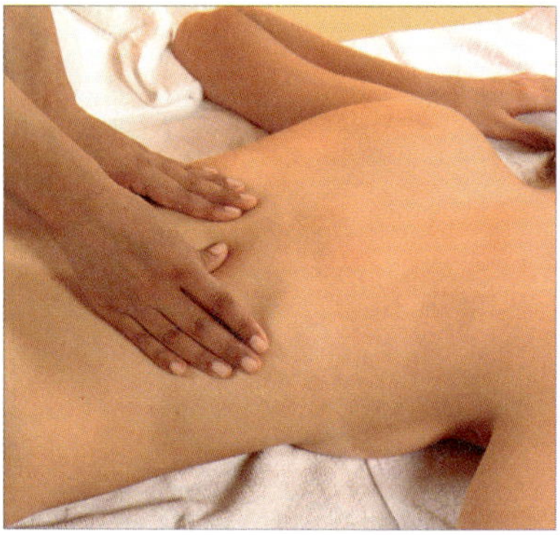

3. With the tips of your thumbs, massage along the spinal column, using kneading motions to relax and relieve tension built up in the back.

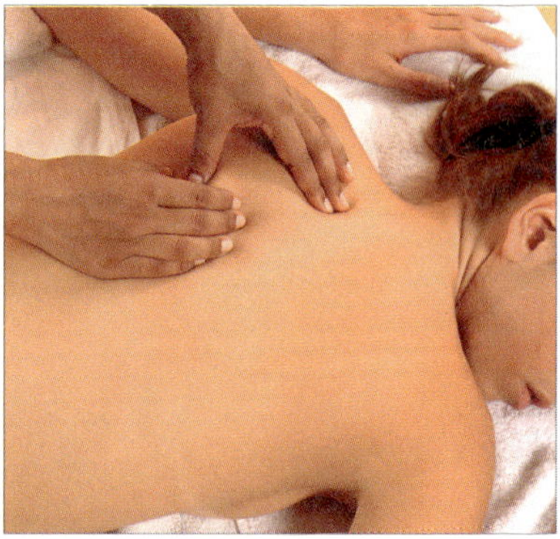

4. Continue using the tips of your fingers on the shoulder blades, to get rid of knots.

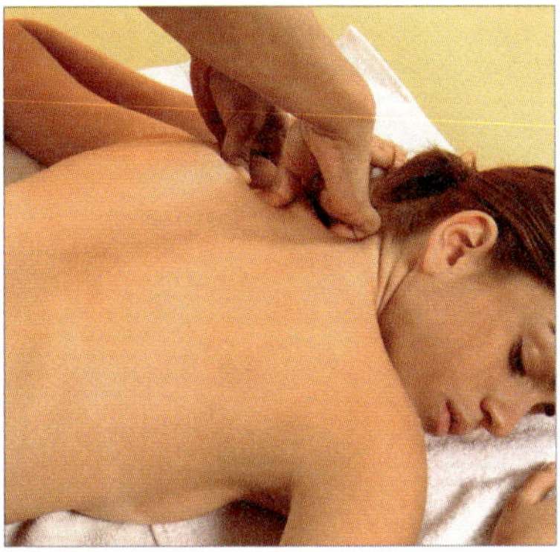

5. *Massage along the back, using gentle pressure to decongest the capillaries.*

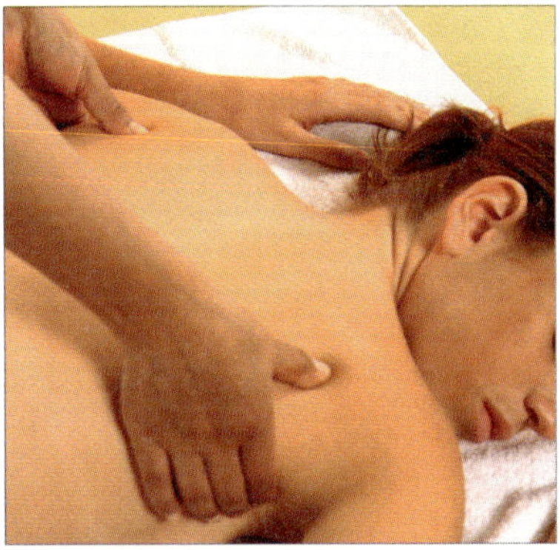

6. *First rubbing motions; next, press with the fingertips of both hands along the shoulder blades.*

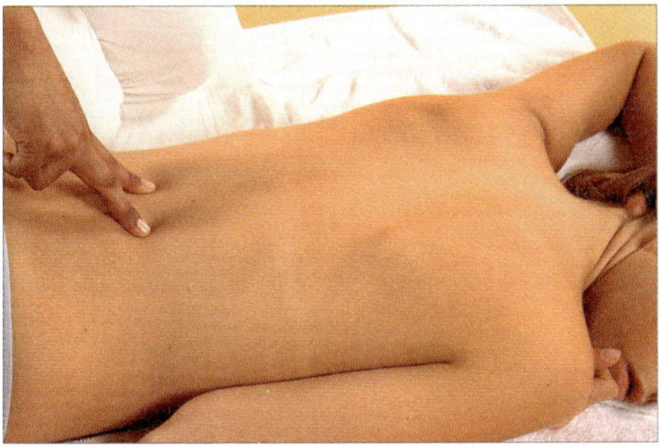

7. *A final relaxing exercise: open your index and middle fingers and run them along the sides of the spinal column. Repeat 20 times.*

BENEFICIAL EFFECTS

These massages can help to bring on sleep because they provide the following benefits that are related to rest:

- **Improve blood circulation and oxygen flow through the blood, which helps to eliminate toxins in the body.**
- **Stimulate the release of endorphins, a substance that helps to bring a sense of well-being and helps to relieve aches and pains.**
- **Reduce stress, fight against depression and low energy.**
- **As with self-massages, relaxing massages can bring more than just physical benefits. When practiced regularly and with dedication, they can move energy to transform the conscience, clear the mind and improve the balance between the body, mind and spirit.**

Calming hydrotherapy

Since ancient times water has been used as a natural medicine to cure the human body. Hydrotherapy is the use of water at different temperatures to revitalize, maintain, and restore health.

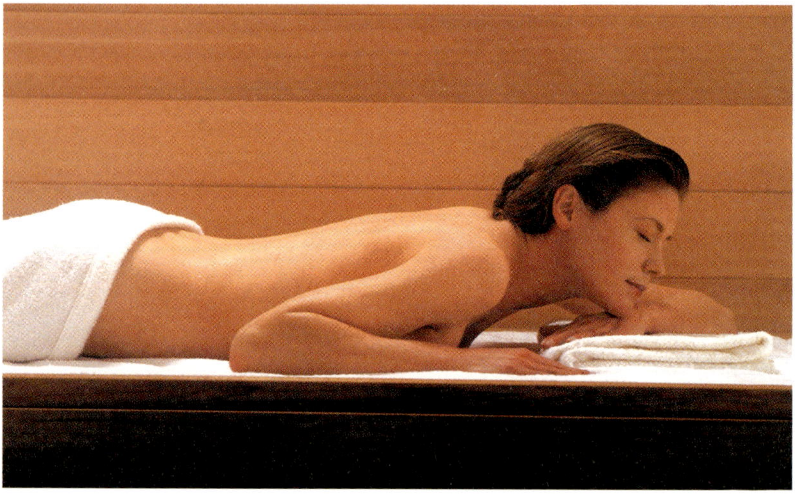

There are a number of hydrotherapy techniques that can be used based on the physical needs of an individual. The most common techniques are those using hot water or vapors for their sedative effects. However, there are techniques using cold water to help fight insomnia.

SPONGE BATH

This is a simple technique that has gained importance for its beneficial effects. The entire body is wet with a washcloth or sponge as fast as possible. Begin with the forehead of the body and then continue from the neck to the base of the feet, rubbing with a sponge soaked in cold water. This therapy helps to calm the nerves and to stimulate the digestive system, favoring better absorption of nutrients and helping to bring on sleep.

COLD WRAPS

A moistened linen cloth is used on different parts of the body, and then covered with a dry woolen cloth to cover up the area. It is used on one part of the body at a time. The most common areas are the chest and abdomen. Chest compresses can be used from the head all the way to the lower back to freshen and decongest the central nerves, bringing a calming and sedative effect. Abdominal compresses are used by covering the lower part of the chest, including the ribs and pelvic bone, which helps to freshen and decongest the digestive system. It also acts as an effective therapy for the stomach, the kidneys and the bladder, getting the body ready for sleep.

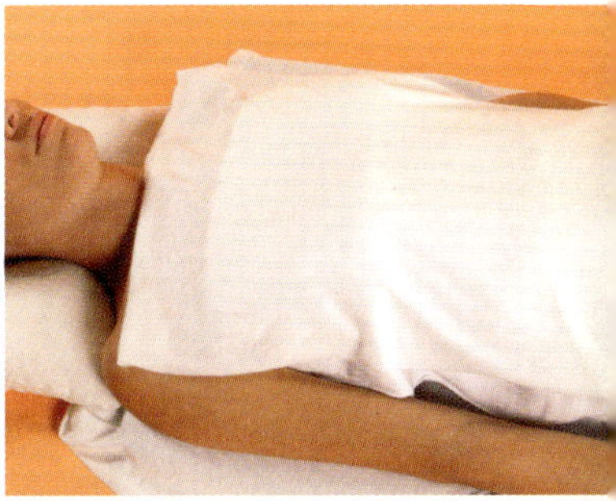

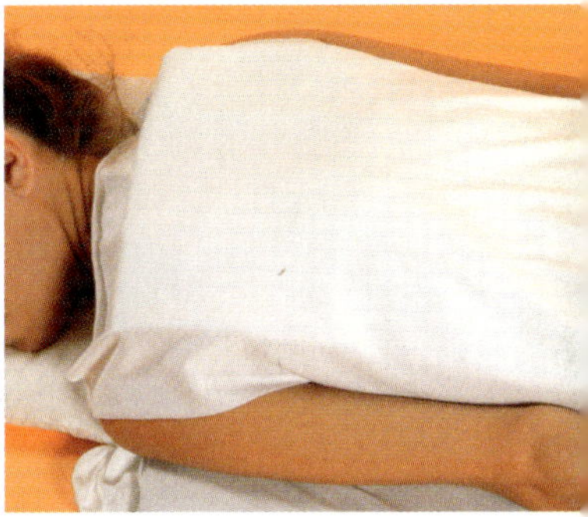

OTHER HYDROTHERAPY TECHNIQUES

- **Watsu.** It *combines water and* shiatsu, *a form of Japanese finger pressure massage applied to the meridians of* chi. *The technique consists of floating in water and supported by the* watsu *practitioner, the* watsu *receiver passes into a state of complete relaxation as gentle stretching is applied to specific areas. More than just a massage, this technique involves a series of free-flowing movements that increase flexibility and strengthen muscles.*
- **Scottish shower.** *This is a type of massage using shower jets to apply pressure. It helps to tone the muscles, it stimulates oxygen flow to the muscle tissues, increases the skin's resistance, stimulates circulation and more than anything helps to rejuvenate your body.*

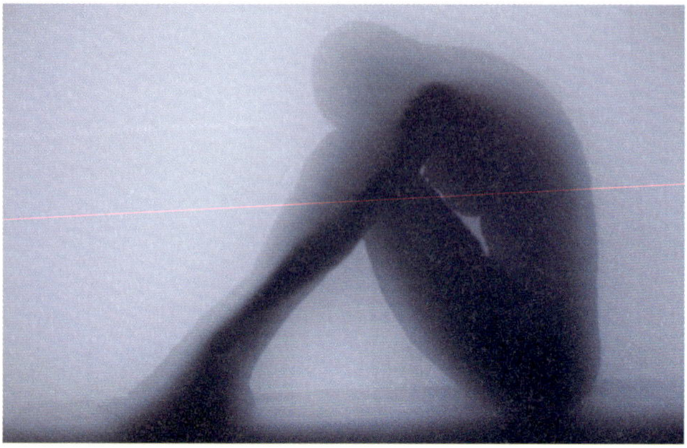

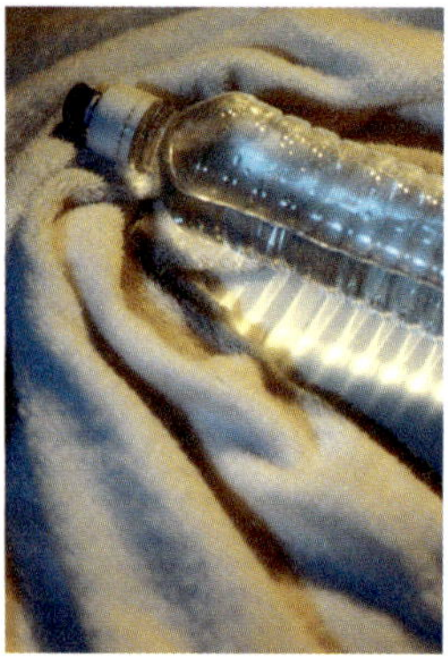

STEAM BATHS

Steam baths are a purifying and tranquilizing therapy. They stimulate the skin and cause sweating which cleans the body from the inside out, making you feel good and relaxed. Steam baths are a good way to fight stress and reduce nervous tension, they can help bring on sleep without any difficulties. Steam baths originated in the ancient Roman Empire and the Arab world: both cultures used thermal baths as a place for relaxation and social meetings. Today, steam baths are used as a treatment to relieve the pressures we find in our everyday lives and to improve our overall physical and mental health. There are different types:

- **Turkish steam bath**, the name comes from its place of origin, Turkey. This type of therapy consists of a series of warm, humid chambers of varying temperatures ranging between 113 °F /45 °C to 158 °F/70 °C. The heat is generated by scorching water that circulates through piping and radiators located on the walls. The humidity is such that the sweat created from the

SAFETY

Steam baths should not be taken by persons with acute infection, high blood pressure, hepatic or renal insufficiency, hyperthyroidism, inflammation of blood vessels (varicose veins, phlebotrombosis) or artherosclerosis. Before taking them, you should consult your doctor.

heat doesn't evaporate. Because of this, the body doesn't get cold and sweats even more.

- **Sauna uses dry heat;** the temperature inside a sauna is generally 140 °F/60 °C, but can be higher than 203 °F/95 °C, depending on your resistance to heat. When you take a sauna you lie down on wood benches, the higher you are the hotter the air. The bath, which shouldn't last for more than 8 minutes, is done in consecutive sessions, separated by 10-minute resting intervals. Because the heat is dryer than a Turkish steam bath, the sweat on the skin dries causing a more pleasant sensation.

- **Finnish bath** consists of sitting in clouds of vapor that are produced by pouring water with essential oils of mint or eucalyptus on porous hot rocks. This steam bath, is a closed room in which temperatures can go up to 113 °F/45 °C.
It helps to purify the respiratory system and relieves tension. It is good for those who are suffering from fatigue and stress. Before taking a Finnish bath it is suggested that you consult your doctor.

IN YOUR ROOM

Hot vapor from a vaporizer with a few drops of essential oil adds to the room's humidity and helps to prevent and relieve congestion, at the same time helping to bring on sleep.

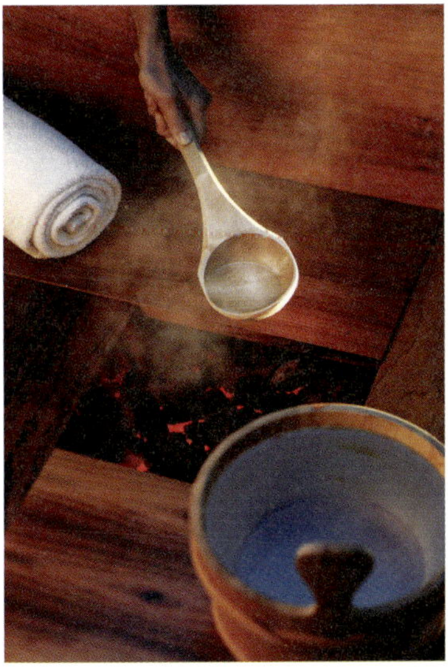

Herbs for natural rest

Nature provides us with a number of plants and products that can be very helpful for treating our health, among those medicinal herbs that help to fight insomnia and its causes. In the following pages, we have developed a guide of the most efficient plants that may work as remedies for insomnia and a list of essential oils from A to Z, that when used topically can help bring on sleep.

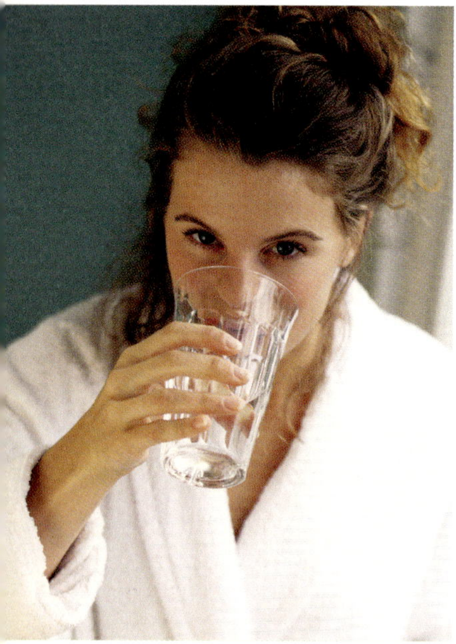

Natural herb remedies make a therapy as old as human civilization. Today, the use of natural herb remedies has been proven scientifically for their therapeutic properties and diverse uses, in powders, grains, capsules, teas or tinctures, salves and gels. Alone or combined with other herbs, many healing plants can be used in cases of insomnia, and they are not as strong as many over-the-counter or prescribed sleep aids. Natural herbal sleep aids do not create dependency. However, before beginning natural herb treatment, it's recommended to see a doctor.

NOTE
You should always consult your physician before starting any herbal treatment.

Red poppy

(Papaverroheas)

- **Parts used.** The petals of the flowers that are cultivated in the summer. They are stored away, conserved and used to make infusions or used as extracts and powders.
- Native to the Far East it is used for its sedative and antispasmodic effects. Red poppy

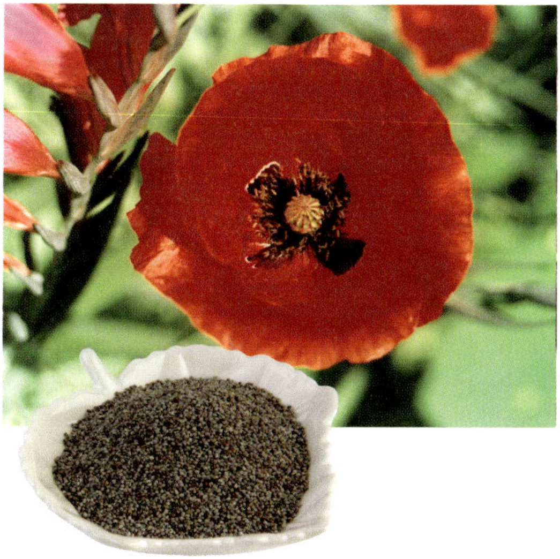

is very useful against anxiety and insomnia. You can take up to 300 mg of dried and ground petals (they are sold in capsules).

• **Warning.** Red poppy should not be administered to small children or pregnant women.

INFUSION FOR CHILDHOOD

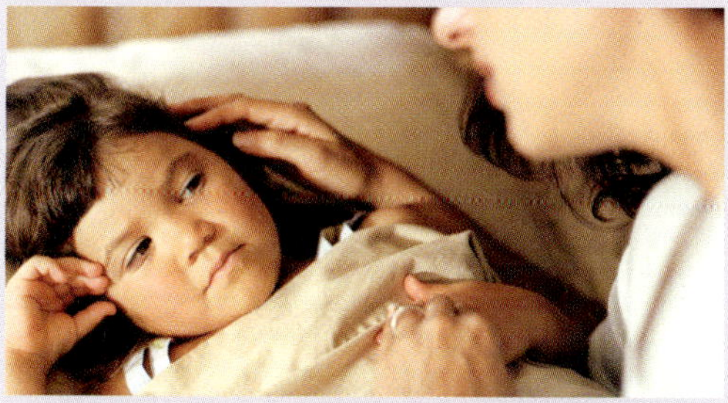

FOR CHILDREN OLDER THAN 5 YEARS OF AGE

Place 1/2 teaspoon of dried red poppy petals in a container with 1 cup of boiling water. Allow to steep for 3 minutes and strain. This infusion can be used up to 3 times a day. It can also be used cold on eyelids for decongestion and eye baths.

ESSENTIAL OILS FROM A TO Z

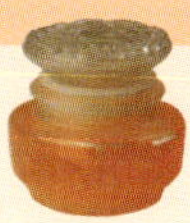

BASIL

The strong, intense aroma of basil can be great for slowing down the mind and getting prepared for sleep. To fight against insomnia, it's suggested to mix basil essential oil with another neutral oil. It can be blended with clary sage, geranium, lavender and lemon balm.

Safety. Basil is not recommended for pregnant women.

BERGAMOT

Perfect for depressive states because it can lift up the spirits through its stimulant and refreshing action.

Safety. Bergamot can irritate sensitive skin. Avoid direct contact with the sun after using it. It mixes well with geranium, juniper, jasmine, lavender, tangerine, neroli, patchouli, camomile, rosemary, marjoram, lemon and ylang ylang.

WARNING

Essential oils are for external use **only**, they should **never** be ingested. Keep stored away from children and keep away from your eyes.

California poppy

(Eschscholtzia californica)

- **Parts used.** The flowers are prepared in infusions and used to make tinctures, syrups, powders and capsules.
- As its name suggests, it is native to California. Today, it is cultivated and used worldwide.
- From the poppy family, California poppy has an active alkaloid compound, that has sedative and painkilling effects. However, it doesn't have any toxic or addictive properties. It is recommended if you are nervous, stressed and suffering from insomnia.
- **Warning.** It can produce side effects during pregnancy, breast-feeding and glaucoma. It's best to take interval breaks from using this treatment (1 week without using this herb for every 40 continuous days of treatment).

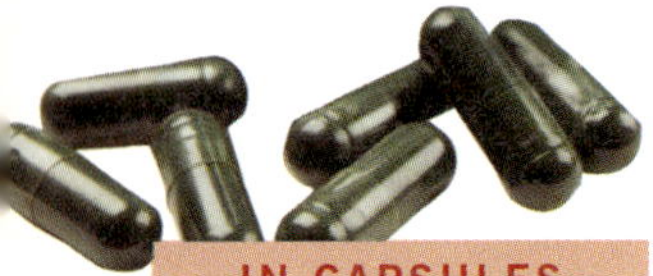

IN CAPSULES

Calming remedy. It is recommended taking 2 capsules a day of California poppy, 30 minutes before each meal. For trouble sleeping, 1 capsule before going to bed.

EFFECTIVE COMBINATION

Infusion to help you sleep well. This infusion is prepared with a base of California poppy, hawthorn and passion flower. Mix 1 tablespoon of each of these herbs and add 1 tablespoon of this herb mixture to 1 cup of water. Prepare the infusion by adding the herbs to boiling water, turn off the heat, set to steep for 3 to 4 minutes and strain. It is used before dinner. You can drink it sweetened with raw sugar or honey.

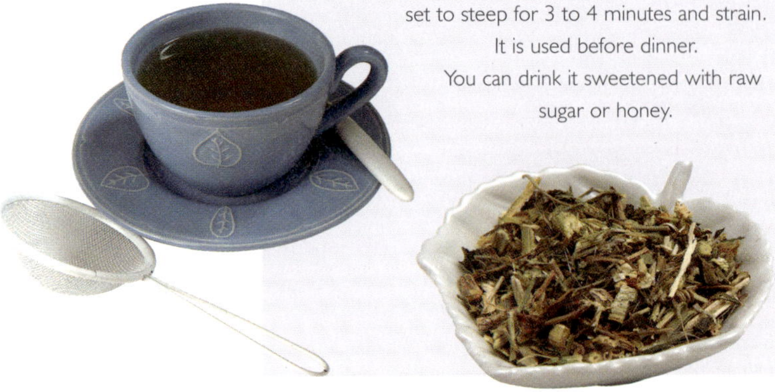

WHAT IS AROMATHERAPY?

Aromatherapy is a holistic remedy that is thought of as a technique to care for the body with the use of essential oils extracted from plants. These oils can stimulate physical, mental and emotional well-being and at the same time they can restore the body's balance and internal harmony. Aromatherapy can be used in massages, compresses, vapors, humidifiers, baths, creams and gargles. Using oils in massage therapy is the most common use because the chemical compounds of the oils are absorbed through the skin, from where they enter the blood flow and produce chemical reactions similar to some medicines. Essential oils should be used under the supervision of a medical professional.

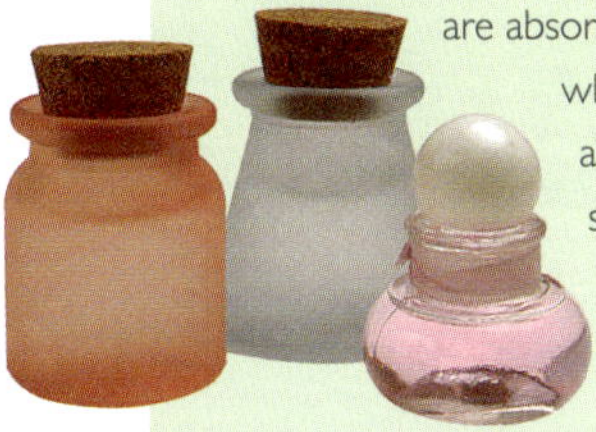

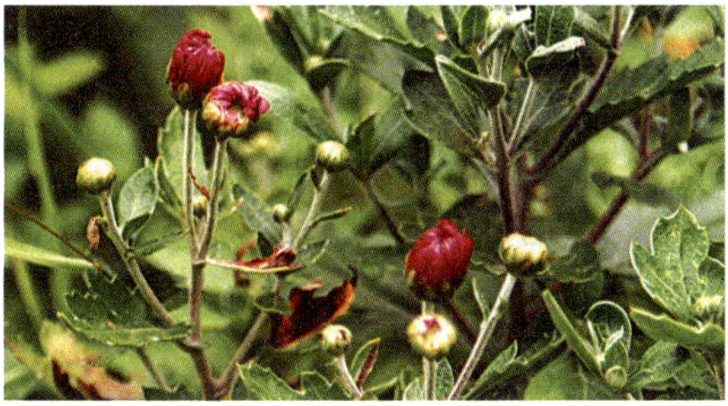

Skullcap

(Scutellaria lateriflora)

- **Parts used.** The aerials (leaves and flowers) are cultivated in the summer. They are used to make infusions, capsules and tinctures.
- Native to North America, the plant has a bitter, almost astringent taste.
- Supports the nervous system and calms stress and anxiety. It has an antispasmodic effect, useful when treating the worries that can cause muscular tension. Ideal for fighting insomnia.

ESSENTIAL OILS FROM A TO Z

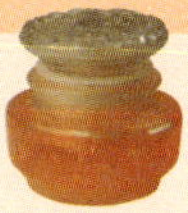

CAMOMILE

Sedative and excellent soothing oil. The herb's sweet fragrance, between floral and fruity, is great for inducing repairing sleep, that helps you get rid of anxiety, anger and fear. It induces a sense of calm and well-being, far away from worries. Combine with bergamot, geranium, jasmine, lavender and ylang ylang.

Safety. It shouldn't be used during the first four months of pregnancy. In large doses it can have an hypnotic effect.

CINNAMON

Recommended for when you feel sad. It has vigorous properties and aids in diverting anxieties before going to bed.

Safety. Do not use during pregnancy, breast-feeding and always use it diluted.

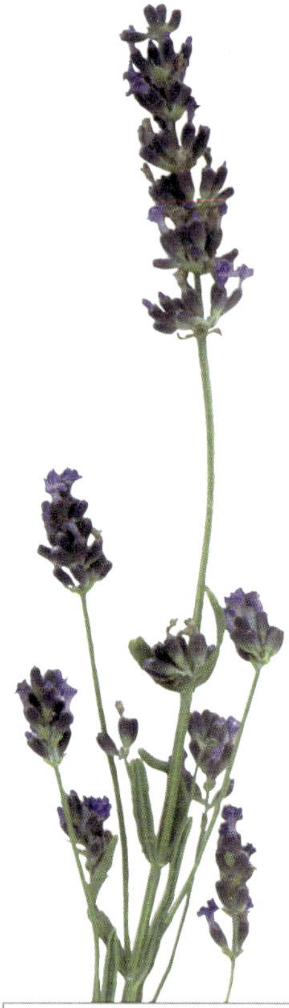

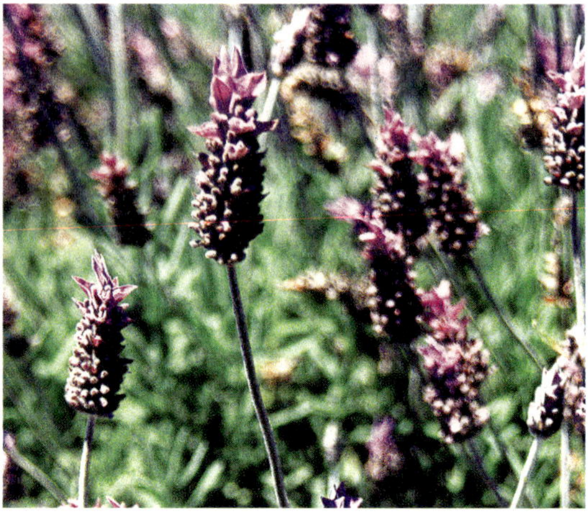

SECRET FOR SLEEPLESS NIGHTS

A little bag of dreams

Prepare a sack of dried hops and place it inside your pillow. Breathing in the herb's aroma will help you sleep better.

Lavender

(Lavandula officinalis)

• **Parts used.** The flowers and to a lesser extent the stems are used to make infusions and decoctions.

• Lavender grows all over Europe and in Northern Africa; also, it's cultivated in a number of countries such as France and the US. It has a strong, pleasant fragrance. The leaves can be added to salads, replacing mint.

• It is used to soothe and promote sleep, helping to relieve heart palpitations and insomnia. It can be taken as an infusion and lavender oil can be rubbed on the skin or used in baths.

Hops

(Humulus lupulus)

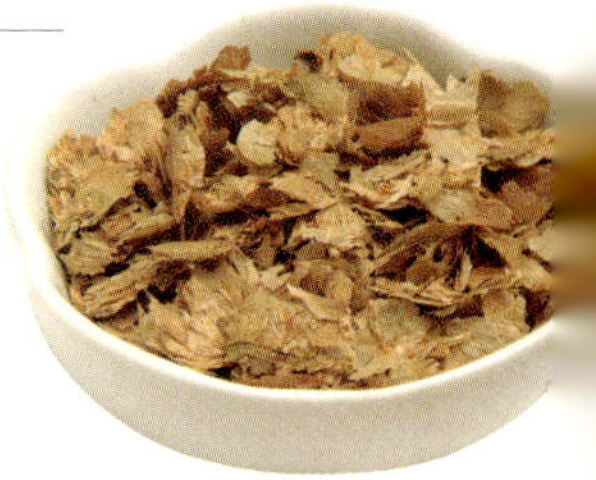

• **Parts used.** Hops are the cone-like, fruiting bodies (strobiles) of the plant and are typically harvested from the cultivated female plants that contain gray

NEUTRAL OILS

These types of oils are used to dilute essential oils for application on the skin. Essential oils should be mixed with a neutral or vehicle oil. It's recommended using grape seed oil and sweet almond oil, which can be found in supermarkets and pharmacies.

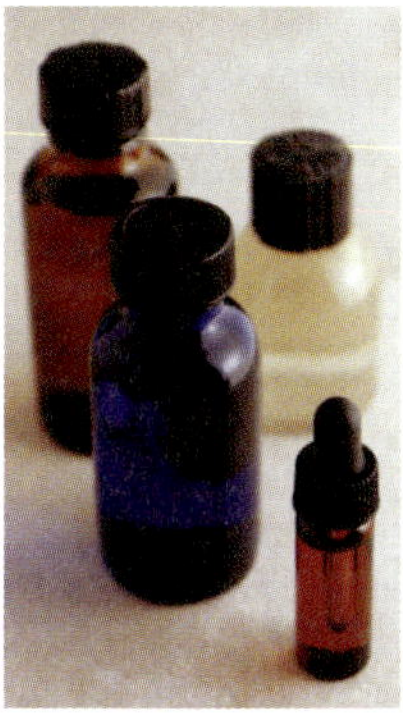

seeds, which are covered with yellow glands. Hops are cultivated in the summer. The fruit can be used to make infusions, liquid extract, syrups, or pills.

- A perennial vine that grows in humid conditions and needs plenty of sun. It grows in abundance in the northern Iberian Peninsula, but is widely cultivated throughout the world. It has a pleasant aroma and has a slightly bitter and spicy taste.
- Hops have been found to have mild sedative properties; fight insomnia, heart palpitations and excessive nervousness. The fruiting bodies are used to flavor beer, it has a bitter taste.

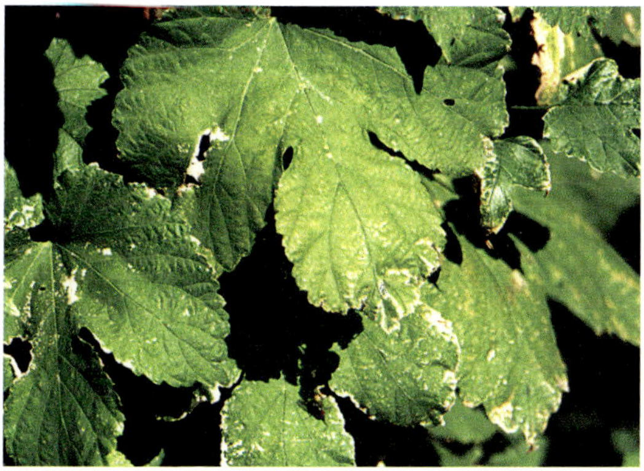

ESSENTIAL OILS FROM A TO Z

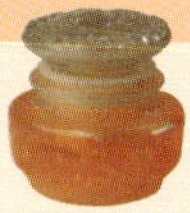

EUCALYPTUS

This essential oil's strong, potent and penetrating aroma helps you to rest and to freshen the air and atmosphere. It can revitalize your energy and reinforce the nervous system. Combine with bergamot, juniper, lemon and rosemary.

Safety. Shouldn't be used if you have high blood pressure or suffer from epilepsy. It should be diluted because eucalyptus can irritate the skin.

INCENSE

This oil can have special soothing properties that stimulate meditation. It is ideal to apply it at night, because it can induce a deep sleep. It slows down breathing, calming and relaxing the mind. With its warm, sweet and penetrating aroma it can create the perfect atmosphere for meditation. It doesn't have side effects. Mix with sandalwood, basil, bergamot and lavender.

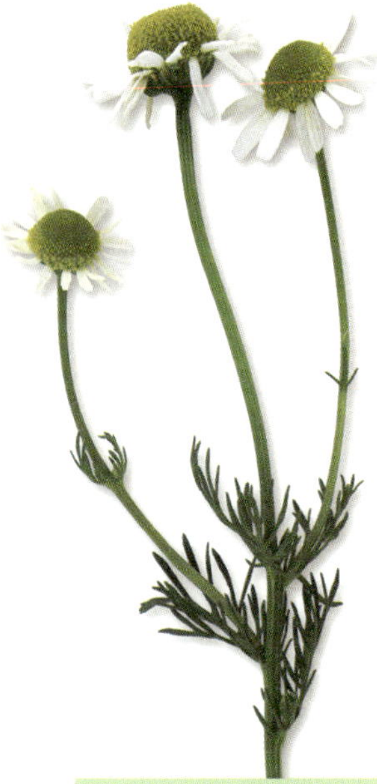

Camomile

(Matricaria recutita L.)

- **Parts used.** The flower-heads or capitula are harvested in the spring. Camomile can be prepared as a tea, using 1 generous spoonful per cup of boiling water. It is also used as a decoction and as tinctures.
- Although this plant is native to Europe, it is also grown in America.
- It calms the nerves and fights muscle spasms; it produces a wonderful soothing effect and aids the digestive system, especially when under stress.
- **Warning.** It doesn't present any side effects, except for those who have allergies or who are sensitive to this plant.

INFUSION TO SLEEP WELL

Make an infusion mixing 1 to 2 teaspoons to 1 cup of boiling water. Set to steep and strain. Drink before going to bed. If camomile doesn't give the desired effect, try linden, lavender or passion flower, which have stronger properties.

Lemon balm

(Melissa officinalis)

- **Parts used.** The leaves are harvested in the summer before the flowers fully blossom and are used (fresh or dried) in a number of ways.

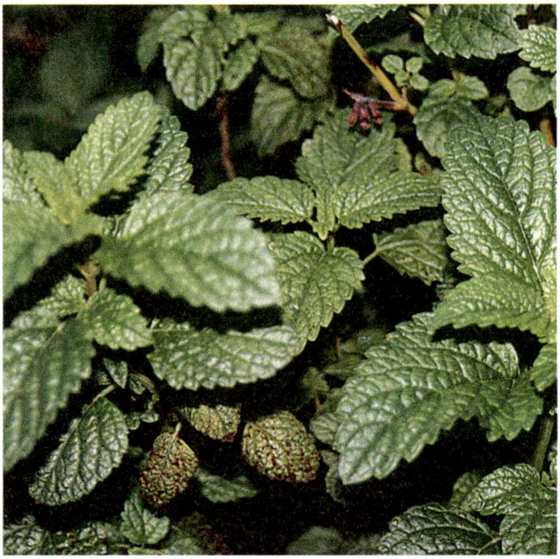

An infusion of fresh lemon balm leaves is a great relaxing tonic. It can be used as a tincture, which is more potent.

- Lemon balm has been used for centuries in Europe, the Far East and Northern Africa and is grown all over the world. It has a slight taste between bitter and sweet.
- It's used as a relaxing tonic that aids to relieve anxiety, slight depression, irritability and digestive problems caused by stress.
- **Warning.** It shouldn't be used if you suffer from hypothyroidism, because lemon balm can alter the level of thyroid hormones.

AROMATHERAPIES

- ***Oils for sleeping.*** *A simple aromatherapy recipe that is effective for helping you sleep well: Place 1/4 cup of distilled water in a spray bottle and add 7 drops of essential oil of lavender and 5 drops of marjoram oil. Spray the face and the sheets as a trick before going to bed.*
- ***Harmonious room.*** *Before going to sleep, its recommended to fill the room with a pleasant aroma with an indicated oil for sleeping, using a heating lamp. Place about 5 to 8 drops of essential oil in a heating lamp and let the oil evaporate.*

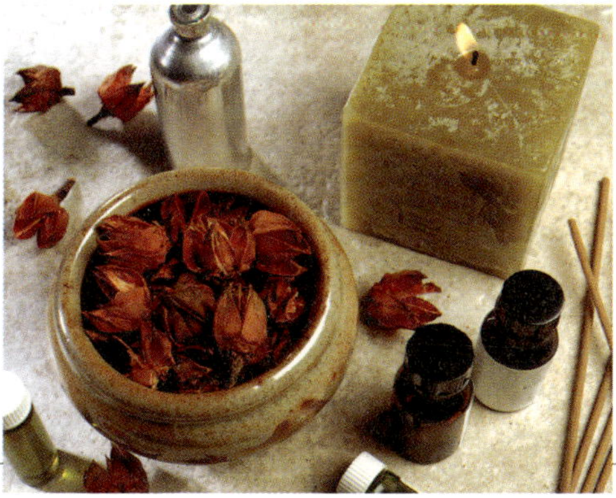

ESSENTIAL OILS FROM A TO Z

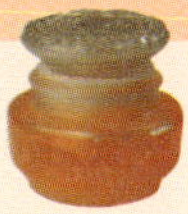

JASMINE

It carries anti-depressive, aphrodisiac, pain relieving and sedative properties. It regulates breathing, calms the nerves and gives a positive, confident outlook.

Safety. It shouldn't be used during pregnancy. However, it can be very beneficial during birth, because it helps to induce contractions and relieves pain.

LAVENDER

Balances the emotions and helps you rest, it also carries pain relieving properties. Its floral and clean aroma (its name comes from the Latin word *lavare*, which means "to clean") which has a regulating effect on the central nervous system and is helpful in cases of exhaustion. Blend with bergamot, camomile, geranium and neroli.

Safety. It shouldn't be used during pregnancy.

Passion flower

(Passiflora coerulea and P. incarnata)

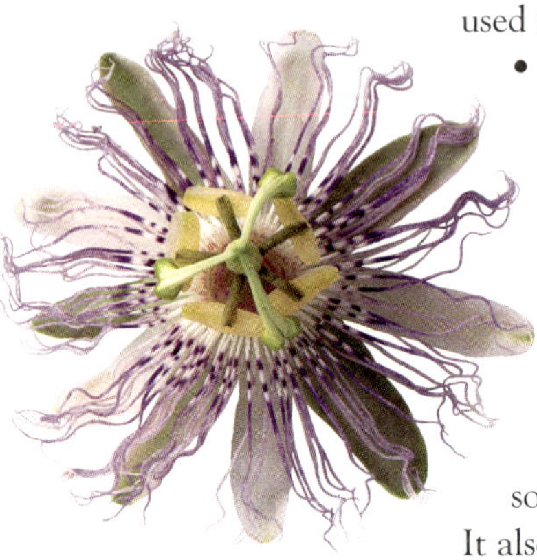

• **Parts used.** The flowers and leaves are used in infusions. The fruit is edible.

• Native to Central America where it's grown most commonly in gardens. A species with similar characteristics, the *Passiflora incarnata*, is grown in Europe.

• Considered to be one of the best remedies against nervous attack, it doesn't have any side effects. Passion flower has sedative and soothing properties, but not depressive. It also makes you sleepy. Ideal for work related stress, mood swings and nervousness brought on by premenstrual syndrome and menopause.

• **Warning.** Do not use passion flower if you are pregnant or breast-feeding. Do not administer to children under 3 years of age. For children under 12 years of age, consult a medical specialist, because the dose should be proportioned to the weight of the child. Eat passion fruit only when very ripe, because the fruit has toxic properties before ripening.

SOOTHING INFUSION

With passion flower. Prepare an infusion with 2 tablespoons of the dried plant in 2 cups of boiling water. Set to steep and strain. Drink a few cups a day.

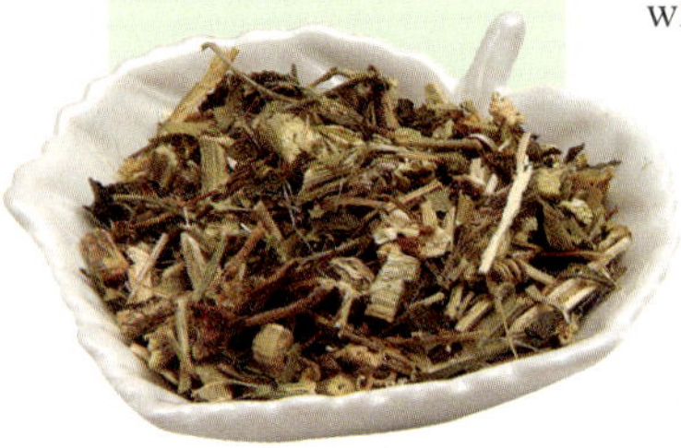

Linden

(Tilia sp.)

• **Parts used.** The flowers, leaves and stems, which can be used as an infusion, as decoction, or to macerate.

• It is also called lime blossom, linden flowers and tilia. It is native to Europe, where it grows in warm climates with clay like soil. It is also found in Asia and North and South America. Although

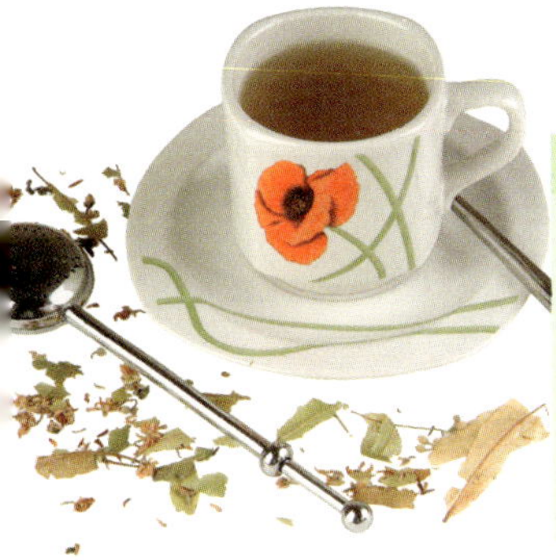

WITH LINDEN

Use 3 teaspoons of dried linden flowers and add to 4 cups of boiling water. Set to steep and strain. Drink when you have symptoms of nervousness.

it prefers to grow in a tropical climate, it also grows in some cold areas of Russia. There are different species which all share similar properties.

- Linden is a relaxing remedy for nervous tension and to soothe the heart and digestive system affected by stress. It has sedative and anti-spasm properties.

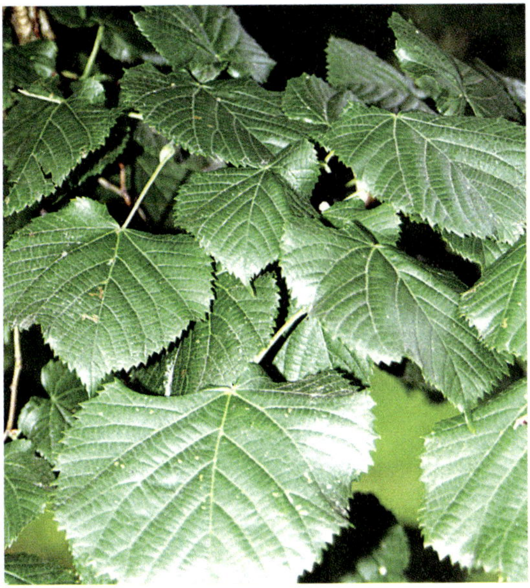

ESSENTIAL OILS FROM A TO Z

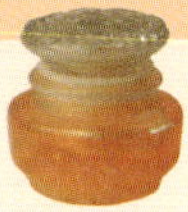

MARJORAM

It can have a calming effect on the central nervous system, reducing hyperactivity and calming anxiety, stress and emotional traumas. However, excessive use can make your mind less alert. It carries painkilling properties and helps to bring on sleep. Its intense herbal fragrance, mixed with almond oil, can work as an anti-depressant. Blend with lavender, camomile and ylang ylang.

Safety. Avoid during pregnancy. It is not advised for small children.

TANGERINE

Tangerine's long lasting, sweet, aromatic and floral aroma calms anxiety and helps depression. It has a hypnotic and calming effect on the central nervous system. It is recommended for pregnant women and children.

Safety. After using tangerine you should avoid exposure to direct sunlight.

Eating well and sleeping better

A balanced diet and regulating the times of your meals, under medical supervision, can be a great help in preventing sleepless nights.

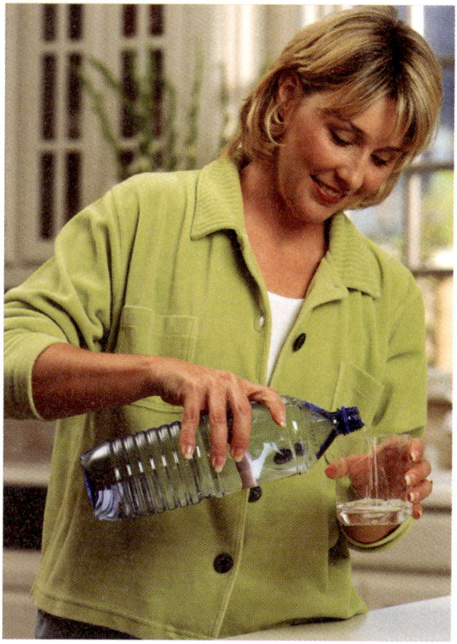

A dinner high in long chain carbohydrates (which your body breaks down slowly) and low in proteins can be helpful in bringing on sleep. Bread, pastas, potatoes and rice can bring effective results. It is also helpful to eat foods containing tryptophan, an essential aminoacid that helps you sleep. Tryptophan is found in **turkey, figs, bananas, dates, yogurt** and **tuna.** Recent studies have shown that Omega-3 fatty acids help you to sleep. **Flaxseeds, sunflower seeds, sesame seeds, pumpkin** and **nuts** all contain Omega-3. Many minerals and vitamins are very important for getting a good rest. We have put together a list with some of the most important nutrients to help you sleep.

AGAINST APNEA

Apnea is obstructived breathing or people who stop breathing repeatedly during their sleep. It can be associated with obesity. To prevent apnea it is important to avoid calorie and fat rich foods like butter, margarine, lard, oils, cakes, cookies and fried foods.

VITAMINS AND MINERALS

Our bodies need vitamins and minerals for specific uses in the body, which our body does not produce. We need an adequate intake of vitamins and minerals in our diets. Those of us who eat a diet lacking essential nutrition tend to get sick often and suffer from insomnia. Studies have proven that foods rich in vitamin C and B complex vitamins and minerals such as calcium and magnesium help to replace energy during sleep. We have compiled a guide to nutrients and their functions and to foods containing that vitamin and/or mineral.

WARNING
You should always consult your doctor before changing your diet.

NOT TOO LITTLE NOR TOO MUCH

One of the golden rules to get a good night's sleep is not going to bed with an empty stomach, because if you are hungry you tend to wake up more. On the other hand, if you want to get a deep, undisturbed night's sleep, you should avoid drinking a lot of liquid at dinner. Excess food is also not advised, because insomnia can be brought on by digestive disorders. It's ideal to eat a light dinner 2 to 3 hours before going to bed.

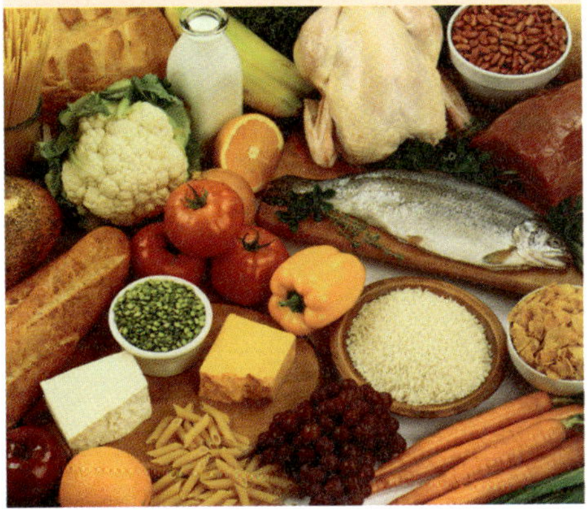

Vitamin B_1

Water-soluble nutrient that the body does not produce, which needs to be incorporated into the diet. Resistant to light, it doesn't break down when exposed to heat. Alcohol, coffee and birth control pills destroy this vitamin. It helps to metabolize carbohydrates and improves digestion. It is an important nutrient that supports the nervous system, fights stress and helps you to rest. Vitamin B_1 deficiency can cause depression and irritability and other symptoms. Foods that are good sources of vitamin B_1 are **wheat germ**, **brewer's yeast**, **whole grain cereals**, **lentils**, **oranges**, **egg yolks** and **nuts**.

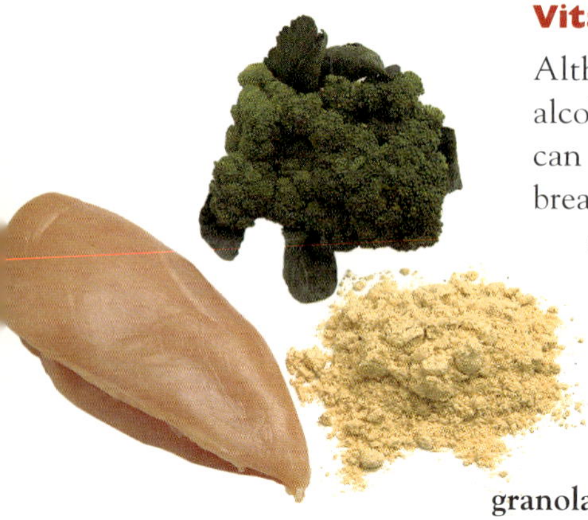

Vitamin B_2

Although it is resistant to heat, alcohol, stress and contraceptive pills can destroy this vitamin. Helps to break down carbohydrates, proteins and fats, as in cellular respiration. It is a fundamental nutrient that supports oxygen flow in the body. It helps you to sleep. It is found in **brewer's yeast**, **cereals**, **granola**, **muesli**, **eggs**, **green vegetables**, **dairy products**, **fish**, **dried fruits**, and **nuts**, like **almonds** and **hazelnuts**.

Vitamin B_3

The aminoacid tryptophan can help synthesize vitamin B_3 inside the human body. It can be exposed to the light, but alcohol, birth control pills and sleeping aids destroy this nutrient. It helps to prevent cardiovascular diseases, reduces cholesterol, and is useful for nervousness like mood swings, paranoia, fear, insecurity, etc. A lack of vitamin B_3 can cause insomnia, because your mind can't calm down and your spirit becomes unstable. As with other B complex vitamins it can be found in **whole grain cereals**, **fish**, **eggs**, **dates**, **figs**, **peanuts**, **almonds** and **brewer's yeast**.

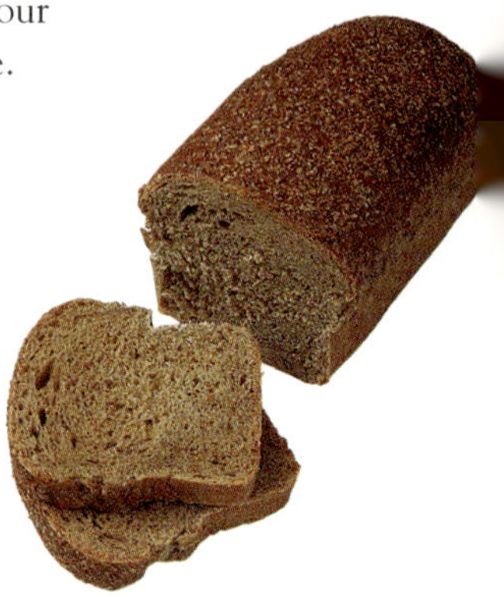

ENERGETIC BREAKFAST

To feel energized and strong all day long it is important to eat a good breakfast in the morning, meaning a healthy and nutritious breakfast. For example: cereal with milk or yogurt, all containing vitamins B_2 and E; fruit juices –like orange juice– that contain vitamin C; seasonal fruits; and even eggs (in an omelette) with fine strips of ham and cheese.

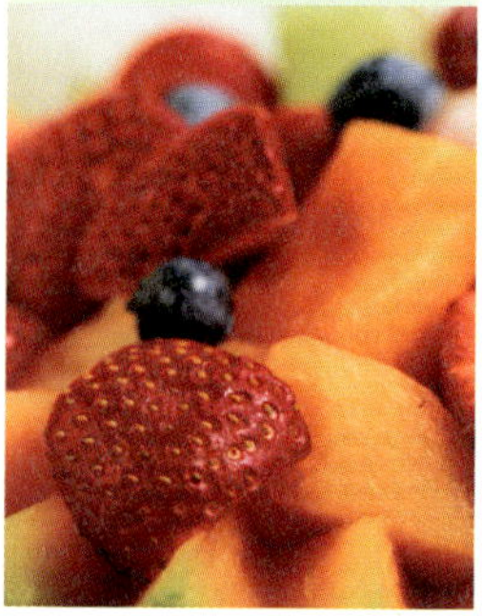

Vitamin B5

The body and intestinal bacteria synthesize this nutrient. It is easily destroyed by alcohol, coffee, birth control pills, sleep aids and cooking. It helps the body break down carbohydrates and proteins. It is helpful in cases of stress and exhaustion. A lack of B5 can cause symptoms such as exhaustion and digestive problems. Good sources of B5 are **meats**, **dairy products**, **eggs**, **brewer's yeast**, **mushrooms**, **whole grain cereals** and **beans**.

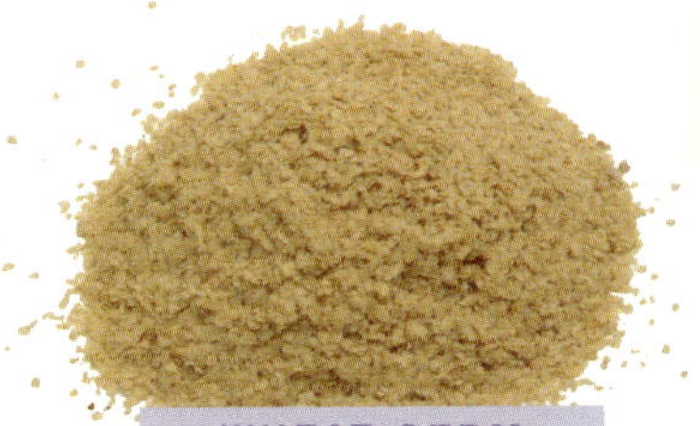

WHEAT GERM

Wheat germ is rich in vitamin B complex, but is also a good source of iron, phosphorus, and vitamin E. It can be very helpful in supporting the nervous system because it contains magnesium, copper and potassium.

Use ground wheat germ added to yogurt, fruit or cereal. You can also add it to salad, soups or stews for an extra nutritious meal.

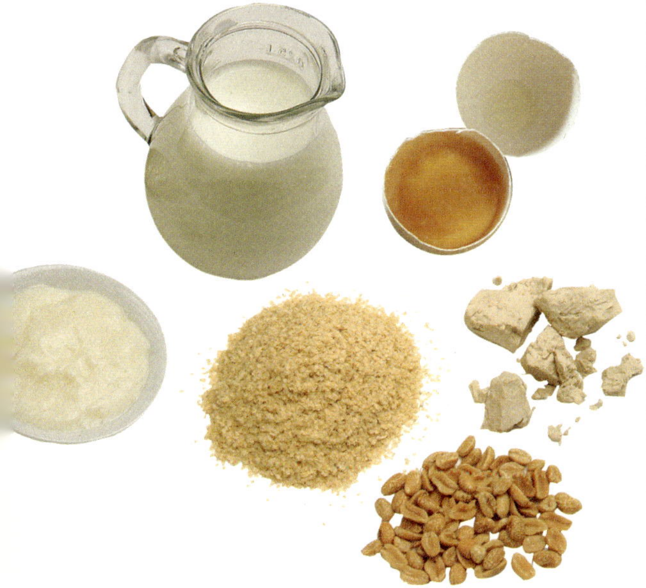

TURKEY

This low-fat white meat is one of the most recommended foods for insomnia because it is rich in tryptophan that helps to bring on sleep.

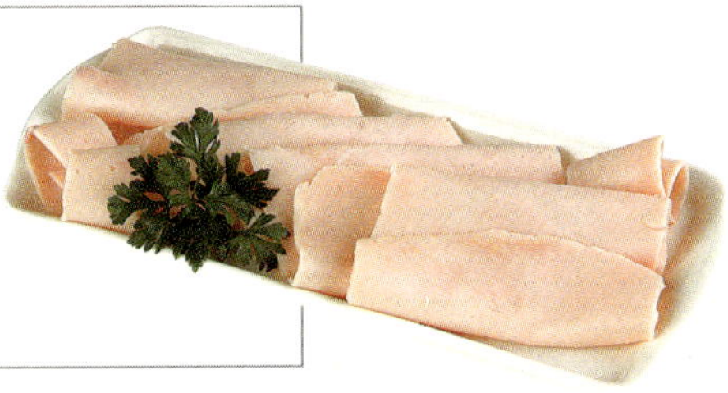

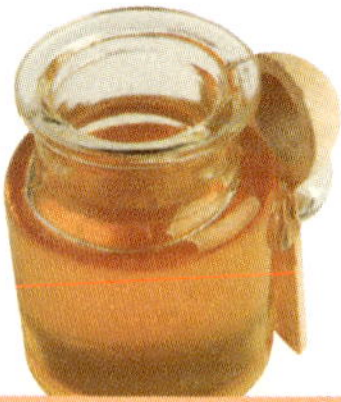

MILK AND HONEY

Vitamins from the B-complex group are found in milk. Also, the aroma and taste of milk brings us back to our childhood. Warm milk with a touch of honey is a comforting beverage, perfect before going to bed. It also provides the body with the calcium and fats that the body needs. It regulates the level of insulin in the body. Insulin released in the body can stimulate tryptophan production and induces serotonin, a neurotransmitter that sends messages between nerve cells and causes feelings of sleepiness. The carbohydrates found in honey also help assimilate tryptophan of milk. You can replace honey with molasses, rich in potassium, copper, iron, calcium, phosphorus, magnesium and vitamins B and C.

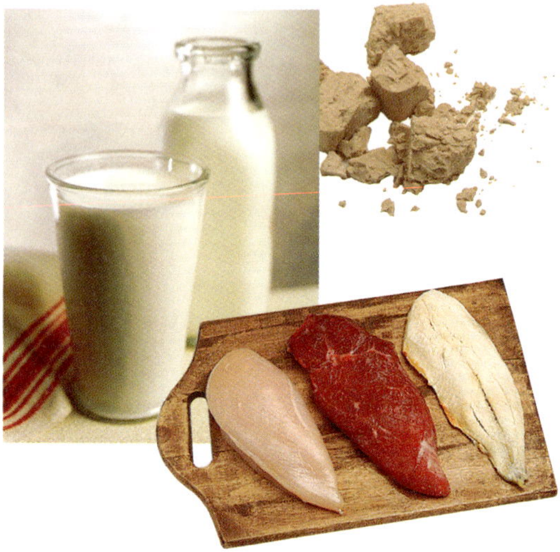

Vitamin B_6

Alcohol and birth control pills break down this nutrient. Meat eaters need a higher amount of B_6 than vegetarians. It is an important vitamin for the immune system. It supports metabolism, especially proteins. It is abundant in natural foods; it is found in **wheat germ**, **brewer's yeast**, **whole grain cereals**, **fish** and **eggs**. A low level of B_6 is associated with insomnia; it's good to include B_6 rich foods such as **pork meat** and **salmon** in your diet.

Vitamin B_8

Supports the body's metabolism of carbohydrates, proteins and fats. It is found in **milk**, **yeast**, **peanuts**, **egg yolk** and **beans**.

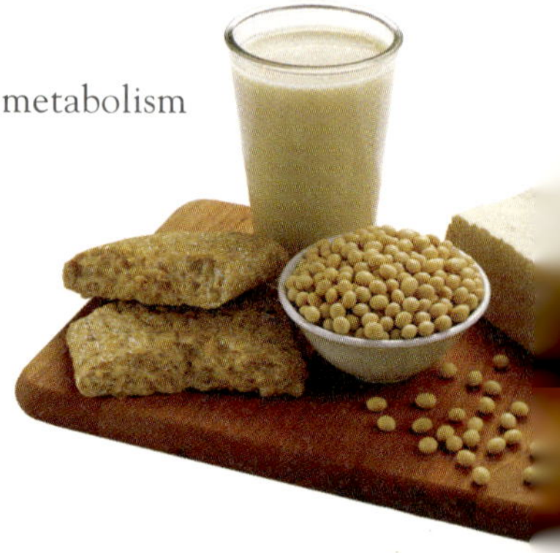

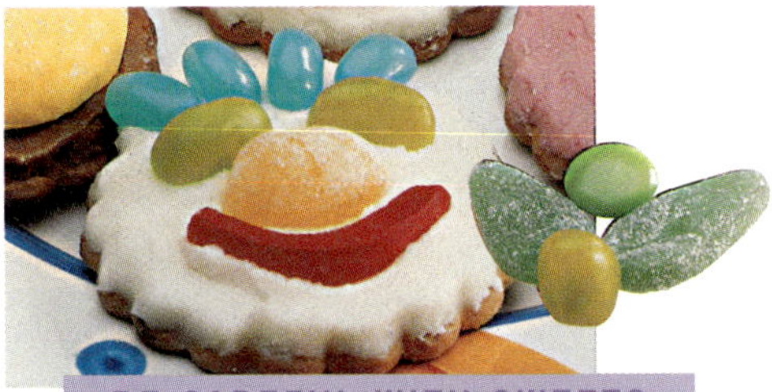

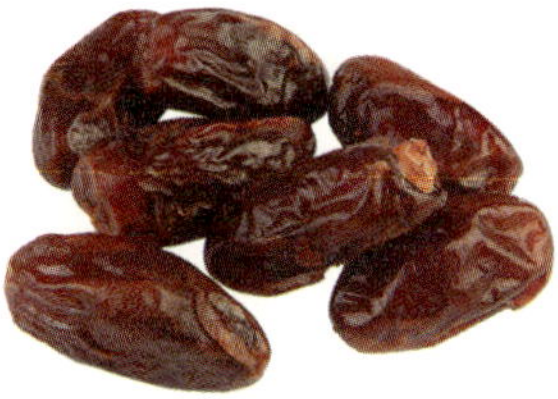

BE CAREFUL WITH SWEETS

It's best to avoid sweets. Sugar, candy, cookies, cakes and soft drinks increase the sugar level in the blood, which is usually followed by "minimal levels".
The foods mentioned above can cause a sense of exhaustion and fatigue, making it difficult to rest well.

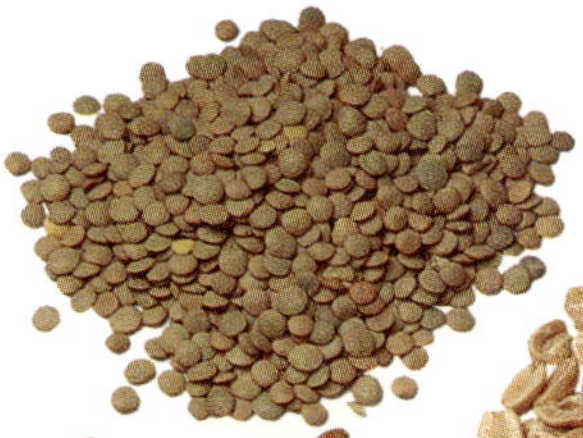

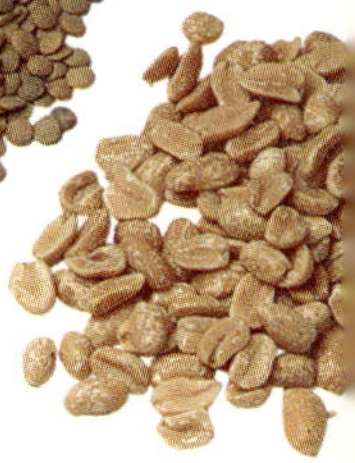

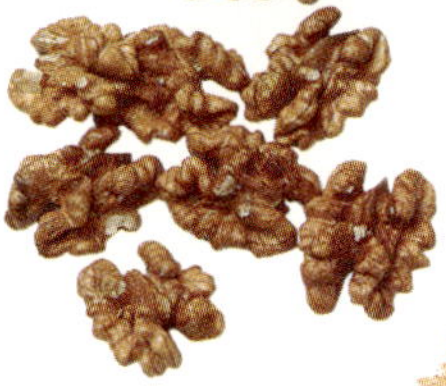

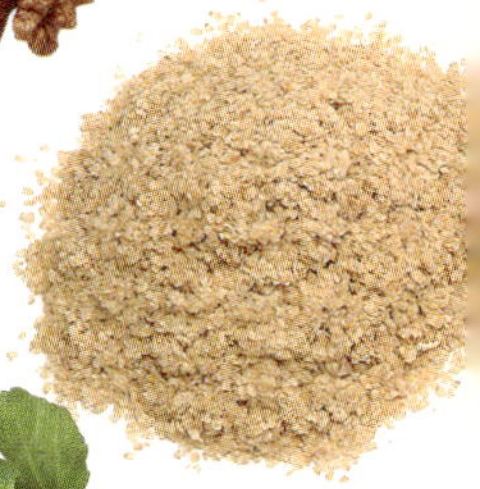

Vitamin B_9 or folic acid

Synthesizes DNA and red blood cells. B_9 deficiency can cause anaemia intestinal parasites and thus, sleeping problems. Some B_9 rich foods: **beans, dried fruits, cabbage, spinach, broccoli** and other **green leafy vegetables, almonds, peanuts** and **brewer's yeast**.

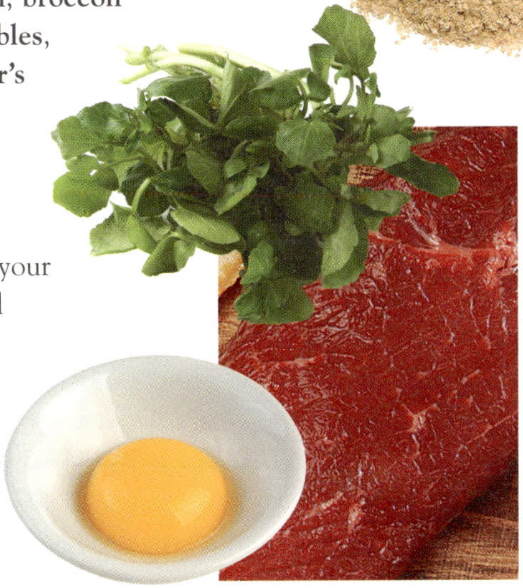

Vitamin B_{11}

Helps to breakdown fats and lowers cholesterol. Increases your energy, muscular stamina and fights against depression and stress.
B_{11} deficiency can result in weak muscles and decreased brain function. It is found in **meats, brewer's yeast, milk, egg yolks** and **oysters**.

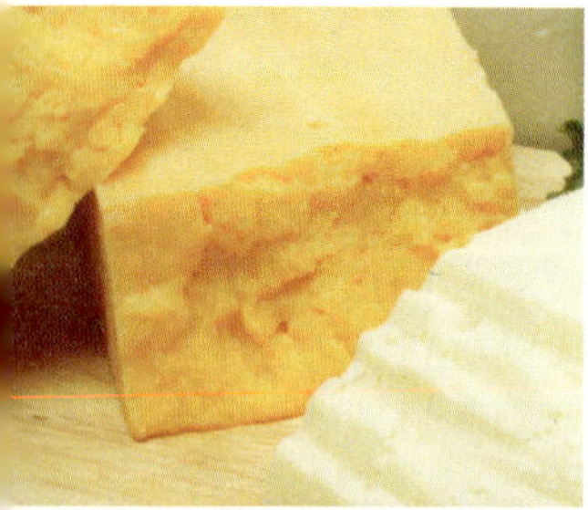

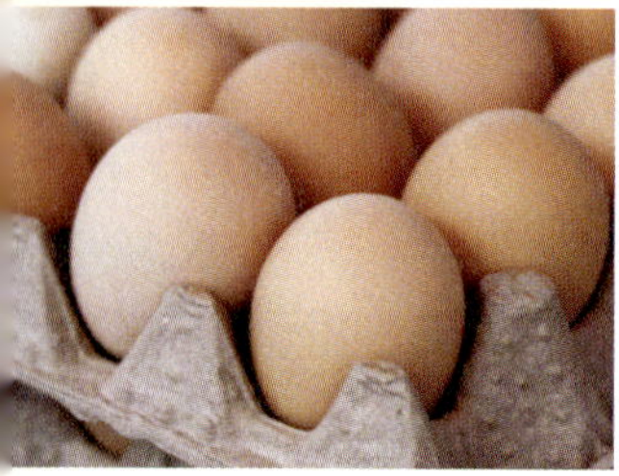

Vitamin B_{12}

A water-soluble vitamin that is destroyed by cooking and light. Alcohol, birth control pills and sleeping pills also destroy it. It forms part of the red blood cells. Prescribed for cases of anaemia because it increases the absorption of iron in the red blood cells. A B_{12} deficiency can cause fatigue and increased nervousness. Found in **meat derived foods**, those who are vegetarian tend to have low levels of vitamin B_{12}. Found in **meats**, **kidney**, **liver**, **dairy** and **eggs**. It is also found in **pollen**, **Spirulina or blue-green algae**, and **brewer's yeast**.

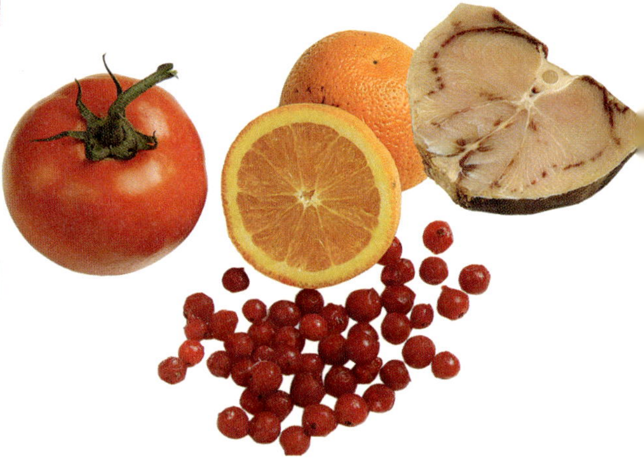

DAILY ROUTINE

Eating at least 2 citrus fruits a day provides an excellent dose of vitamin C. To make sure your body gets enough vitamin C, it's key to drink a glass of fruit juice everyday.

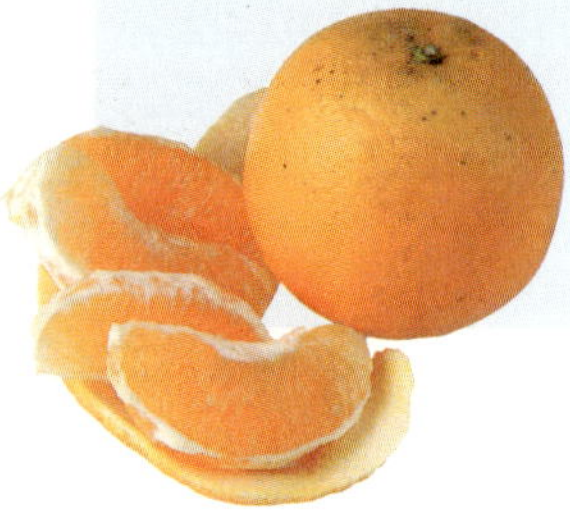

Vitamin C

Is a water-soluble vitamin that is destroyed by cooking, tobacco and aspirins. It supports the immune system and is very beneficial for the body. Vitamin C deficiency can cause susceptibility to infectious diseases, like colds, and causes a number of physical problems, including insomnia. Found in **citrus fruits**, **guavas**, **kiwi**, **green leafy vegetables**, **tomatoes**, **cauliflower** and **sweet potatoes**.

LETTUCE

Green leafy lettuce has a high amount of calcium, which is helpful in bringing on sleep. And the potassium found in lettuce is a fundamental nutrient for the nervous system.

To sleep well: boil 1 or 2 lettuce leaves for five minutes in 2 cups of water. Allow to cool and filter. Sweeten the mixture and drink 1 cup 1/2 hour before going to bed. Do not drink this infusion if you have bile duct problems.

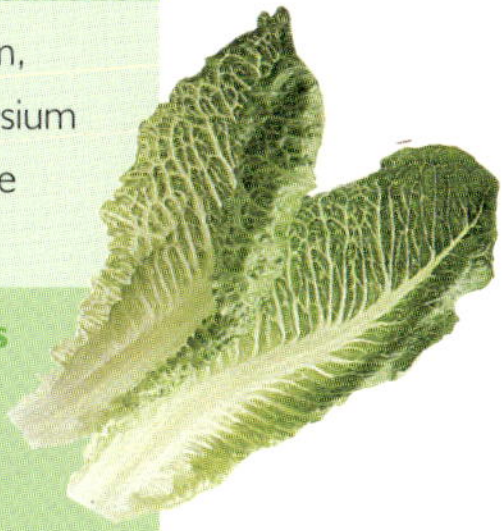

Calcium

99 percent of calcium in the body is found in the bones and teeth, the remaining 1 percent circulates in the tissues and body fluids. This mineral is important for the coagulation of the blood and for heart muscle contractions. It is also an essential mineral for the transmission of nerve signals. A deficit can result in cramping, spasms, slow pulse, heart palpitations and insomnia. Calcium is found in **dairy products**, **sesame seeds**, **sunflower seeds**, **almonds**, **hazelnuts** and other **nuts**, **algae** and **fresh vegetables**.

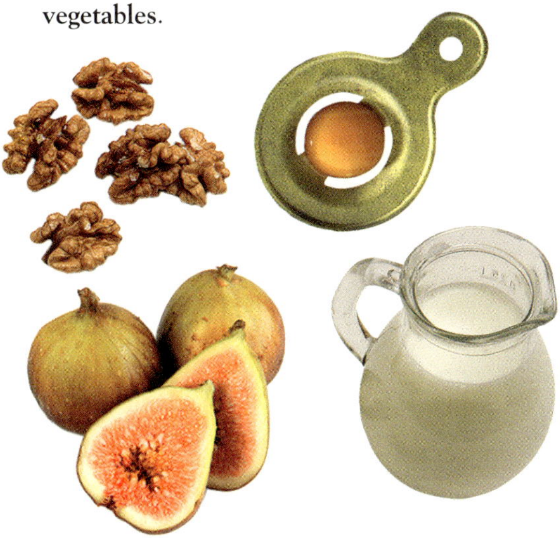

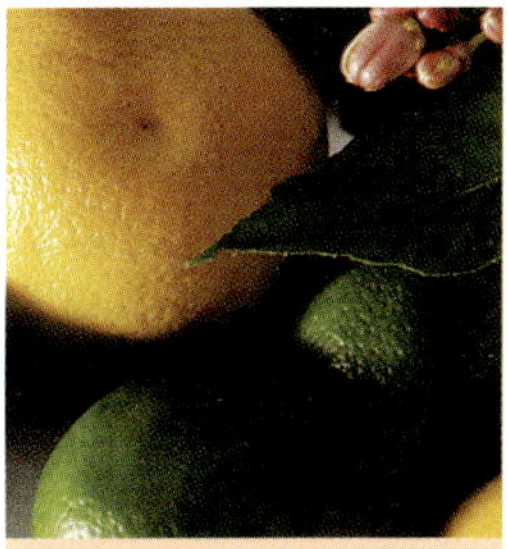

TO ENSURE IRON ABSORPTION

Fruit juices –like orange, lime and grapefruit juices– increase the absorption of iron, while coffee and cafeinated teas have the opposite effect, they impede iron absorption. It's good to use lemon juice to dress salads and to flavor foods, it's also good to accompany meals with lemonade. Avoid drinking tea and coffee after lunch and dinner.

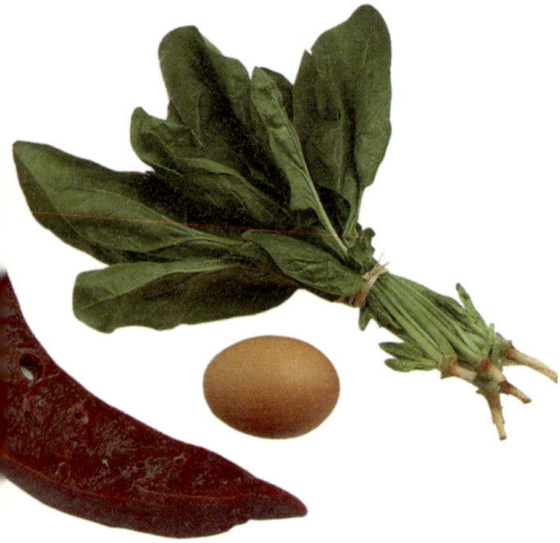

Iron

Iron is found in the body's red blood cells and is fundamental for the formation of hemoglobin, a protein that transports oxygen. It supports the breathing of the body's cells. When the body lacks this mineral, anaemia can result along with lower immunity to illnesses, fatigue and low energy. Deficiency can also cause insomnia. The principal food sources for iron are **red** and **white meats**, **beans**, **dried fruits**, **raisins**, **lentils**, **sunflower seeds** and **green leafy vegetables** like dandelions, spinach and kale.

SLEEPY TEA

with sunflower seeds

In 4 cups of water boil 1 tablespoon of sunflower seeds. Allow to cool, strain and sweeten with a touch of honey. This tea relieves the day's tensions and helps you sleep better. Drink a tepid cup of this tea 1/2 hour before going bed.

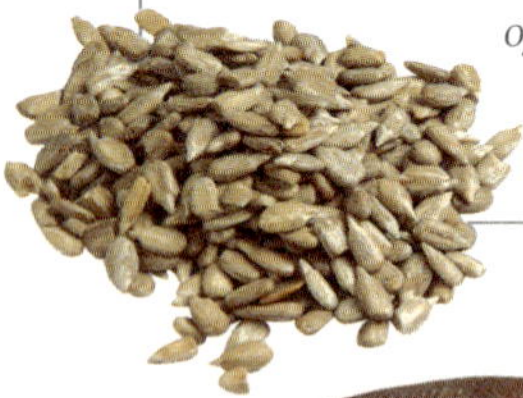

Magnesium

Plays an essential role in developing muscle mass and improving cardiovascular health. Activates enzymes and stabilizes the body's molecules. It acts hand in hand with calcium and phosphorus. Almost 70 percent of magnesium inside the body is found in the bones, the remaining 30 percent is found in the blood and tissues (the muscular system has more magnesium than calcium).
A deficiency can cause irritability, stress and insomnia. Deficiency is common in people who are on long term diets. **Dried fruits** is particularly rich in magnesium, other foods rich in this nutrient include, **almonds**, **soy**, **oatmeal**, **figs** and **dates**.

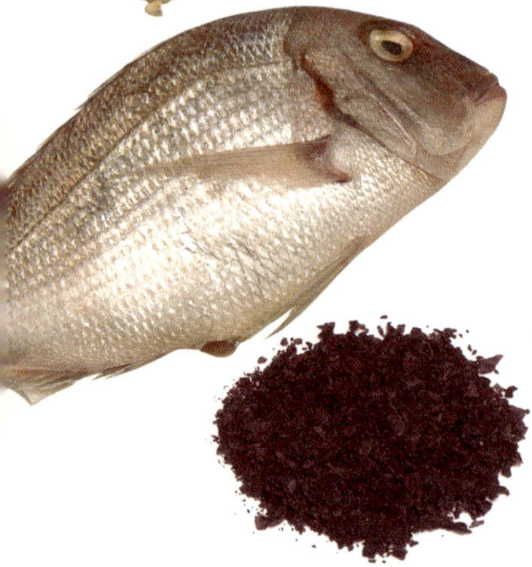

ABC OF EATING AND SLEEPING WELL

It's good to change your meal schedule (breakfast, lunch, snacks and dinner), according to the same number of hours that your waking time has changed. That's to say, if you are waking up earlier than usual and going to bed later, you should eat breakfast and the rest of your meals earlier, eating dinner the same number of hours earlier than you have woken up.

- **Breakfast** should be the most important meal of the day, rich in vitamins, protein and calories.
- **At mid-morning** you should eat a small snack, which could be a yogurt, seasonal fruits, flavored gelatin or stock (in the winter).
- **Lunch** should be rich in proteins (beef, poultry, fish or pork) and seasonal vegetables.
- You should not skip your afternoon snack, it's suggested eating a yogurt or fruit. Whenever possible, try to avoid drinking cafeinated drinks after midday.
- **Dinner** should be light, try and avoid oils, fats, high proteins and other foods that require complex digestion. You can choose between a plate of pasta, rice with a hard boiled egg, fruits, jam or cream cheese with bread.
- **Alcoholic drinks** can be deceiving, making you think that they make you sleepy, when on the contrary they keep you from sleeping soundly.

OATMEAL

For pregnant women

Oatmeal has sedative, diuretic, mineral and antioxidant properties. This grain has a number of gentle effects for pregnant women who are having trouble sleeping or temporary nervousness. It is recommended to eat a bowl of oatmeal a day or to take 1 teaspoon of oatmeal tincture diluted in water 3 times a day.

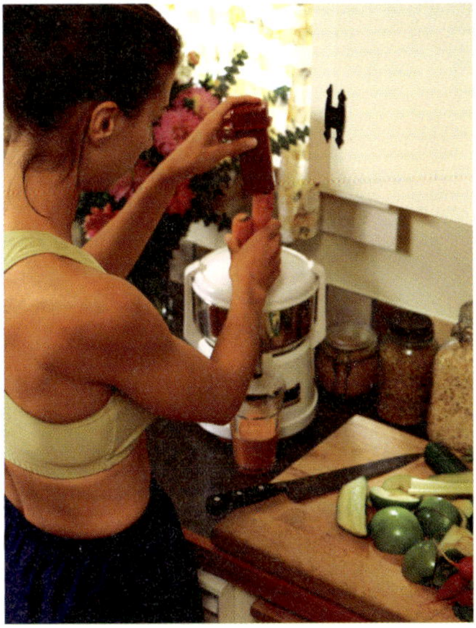

Sleepy diet for an energized life

A diet rich in tryptophan can improve your sleep. Tryptophan is an aminoacid that is a major building block for making serotonin, a neurotransmitter which sends messages between nerve cells and causes feelings of sleepiness.

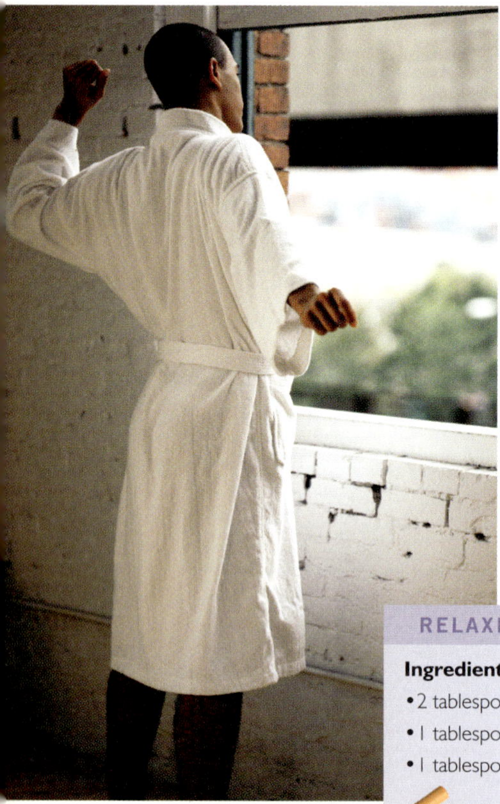

For tryptophan to be effective in improving sleep, it's suggested eating between 1 to 5mg a day. This amino acid is abundant in whole grain cereals, turkey, tuna, bananas and plantains, dates, dried figs, nuts, yogurt and milk.

We have put together a suggested complete menu, during the entire week, comprised of specific foods that aid in improving your sleep.

RELAXING INFUSION WITH HONEY

Ingredients

- 2 tablespoons of hops flowers
- 1 tablespoon lemon blossom
- 1 tablespoon of hawthorn

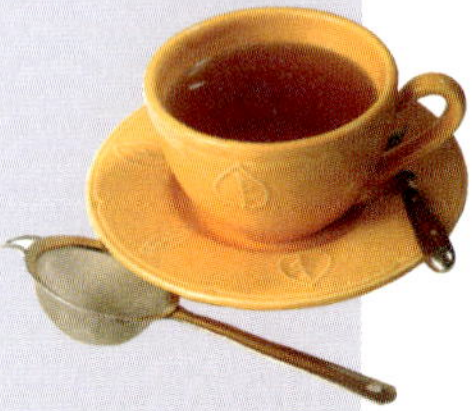

Preparation

Place in 1 cup 1 spoonful of this mixture, fill the cup with boiling water, allow to steep, covered, for 15 minutes and strain. Sweeten with honey and drink tepid.

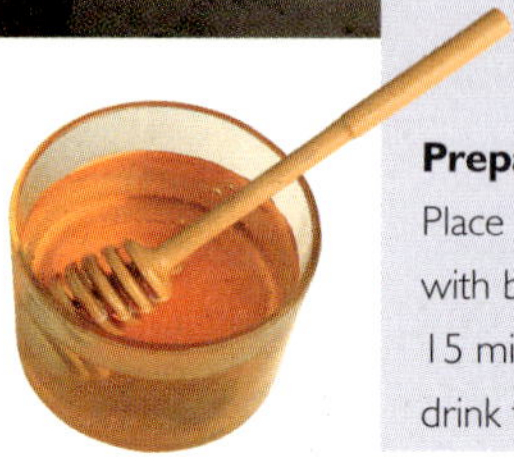

MONDAY	TUESDAY	WEDNESDAY
BREAKFAST • *1 glass of orange juice with 3 teaspoons of brewer's yeast and 3 drops of wheat germ oil* • *1 glass of skim milk with 1 teaspoon of decaf instant coffee.* • *2 slices of wholewheat bread* • *1 teaspoon of honey*	**BREAKFAST** • *1 glass of orange juice with 3 teaspoons of brewer's yeast and 3 drops of wheat germ oil* • *1 glass of skim milk* • *2 slices of wholewheat bread with 2 teaspoons of plum jam*	**BREAKFAST** • *1 glass of orange juice with 3 teaspoons of brewer's yeast and 3 drops of wheat germ oil* • *1 glass of skim milk* • *2 oz/ 60g of muesli*
LUNCH • *Whole grain rice with spinach* • *Tomato and celery salad* • *6 oz/180 g of lean pork*	**LUNCH** • *1 soy burger* • *5 oz/150 g sautéed or steamed spinach* • *Potato, carrot and snow pea salad* • *2 slices of wholewheat bread*	**LUNCH** • *Grilled chicken with leeks, red peppers and beet.* • *1 slice of wholewheat bread* • *1 fruit*
SNACK • *5 walnuts* • *1 cup low-fat yogurt*	**SNACK** • *1 cup low-fat yogurt*	**SNACK** • *1 1/2 oz/ 45 g of dates* • *1 slice wholewheat bread* • *Skim milk with malt*
DINNER • *1 cup of vegetable stock with 1 spoonful of brewer's yeast and wheat germ* • *Lettuce, soybean sprouts and fennel salad* • *2 slices of wholewheat bread* • *1 pear* • *Relaxing infusion with honey**	**DINNER** • *1 cup of vegetable stock with 1 spoonful of brewer's yeast and wheat germ* • *Zucchini scramble* • *2 slices of wholewheat bread* • *Relaxing infusion with honey**	**DINNER** • *1 cup of vegetable stock with 1 spoonful of brewer's yeast and wheat germ* • *Eggplant flan with sweet beet salad* • *2 slices of wholewheat bread* • *Relaxing infusion with honey**

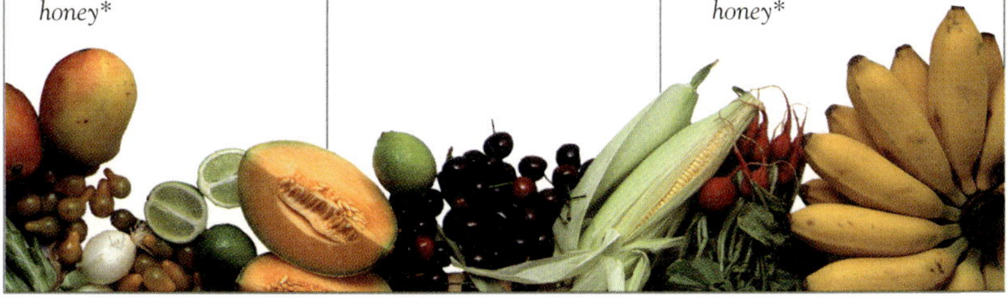

THURSDAY	FRIDAY	SATURDAY
BREAKFAST • 1 glass of orange juice with 3 teaspoons of brewer's yeast and 3 drops of wheat germ oil • 1 glass of skim milk • 3 whole grain crackers	**BREAKFAST** • 1 glass of orange juice with 3 teaspoons of brewer's yeast and 3 drops of wheat germ oil • 1 glass of skim milk with 1 teaspoon decaf coffee or malt • 2 slices of wholewheat bread	**BREAKFAST** • 1 glass of orange juice with 3 teaspoons of brewer's yeast and 3 drops of wheat germ oil • 1 glass of skim milk with 1/2 cup of cereals
LUNCH • Pumpkin and potato purée • 7 oz/ 200 g grilled fish • Lettuce salad	**LUNCH** • Tuna, potato, lettuce, carrot, sweet beet and red pepper salad • 1 fruit	**LUNCH** • 5 oz/150 g of turkey • Fresh basil and tomato salad with fresh mozzarella • 2 slices of wholewheat bread
SNACK • 1 banana • 2 slices of wholewheat bread	**SNACK** • 5 dried figs • 2 slices of wholewheat bread	**SNACK** • 1 cup low-fat yogurt • 2 slices of wholewheat bread
DINNER • 1 cup of vegetable stock with 1 spoonful of brewer's yeast and wheat germ • Pasta with sautéed broccoli • 2 slices of wholewheat bread • Relaxing infusion with honey*	**DINNER** • 1 cup of vegetable stock with 1 spoonful of brewer's yeast and wheat germ • Mixed steamed vegetables with 1 cup of brown rice • 2 slices of wholewheat bread • Relaxing infusion with honey*	**DINNER** • 1 cup of vegetable stock with 1 spoonful of brewer's yeast and wheat germ • Spinach flan with pumpkin purée • Pear compote • Relaxing infusion with honey*

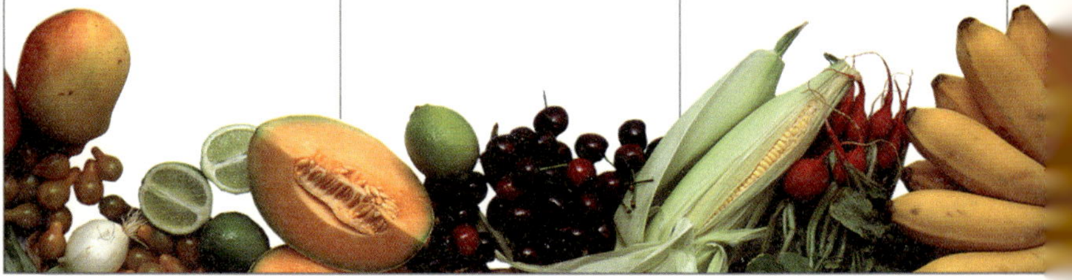

SUNDAY

BREAKFAST

- *1 glass of orange juice with 3 teaspoons of brewer's yeast and 3 drops of wheat germ oil*
- *1 glass of skim milk*
- *2 slices of wholewheat bread*

LUNCH

- *Grilled fish with mixed steamed vegetables*
- *Apple compote*
- *1 slice of wholewheat bread*

SNACK

- *Fruit salad*

DINNER

- *1 cup of vegetable stock with 1 spoonful of brewer's yeast and wheat germ*
- *Chicory with nuts and yogurt sauce*
- *Golden nuggets filled with corn cream*
- *2 slices of wholewheat bread*
- *Relaxing infusion with honey**

* *see* Relaxing infusion with honey *box.*

MACKEREL, SALMON AND SARDINES

These blue fish are rich in Omega-3 fatty acids, which fortify the nervous system and support brain health and the nerves. Eating these fish daily can improve the body's resistance to tensions; in addition they are highly nutritious foods.

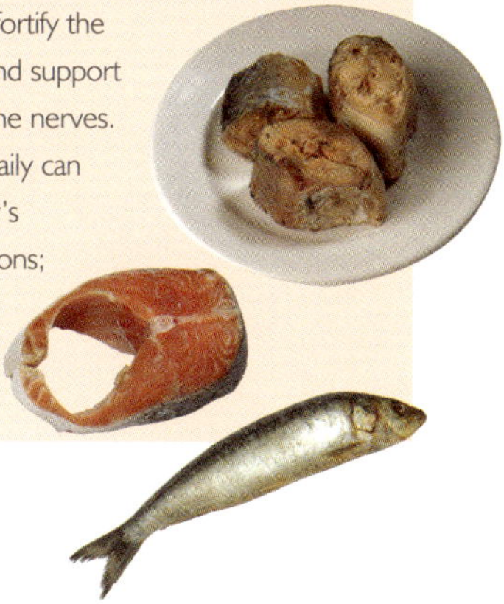

FRUITS THAT HELP YOU SLEEP

Figs, bananas and dates are rich in tryptophan, a substance that can contribute to sleeping. They make a great dessert after dinner, to make sure you get a restful night's sleep.

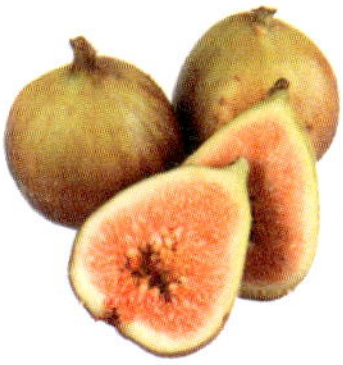

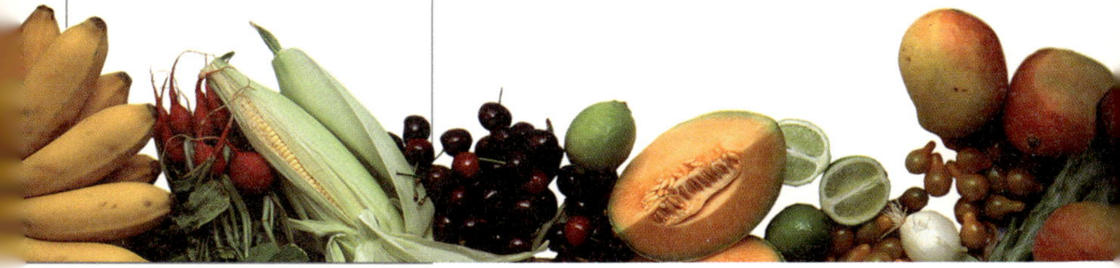

index

Introduction

What is insomnia? 4
What causes insomnia? 6
Changing your lifestyle 8

Complementary Therapies

Visualizing to relax 12
Meditating for a good night sleep 14
Improving your rest with yoga 16
Do-in and… get ready to relax! 20
Reflexes and well-being 32
Restful massages 34
Calming hydrotherapy 36

Natural Herb Remedies

Herbs for natural rest 40

Healing Foods

Eating well and sleeping better 50
Sleepy diet for an energized life 60

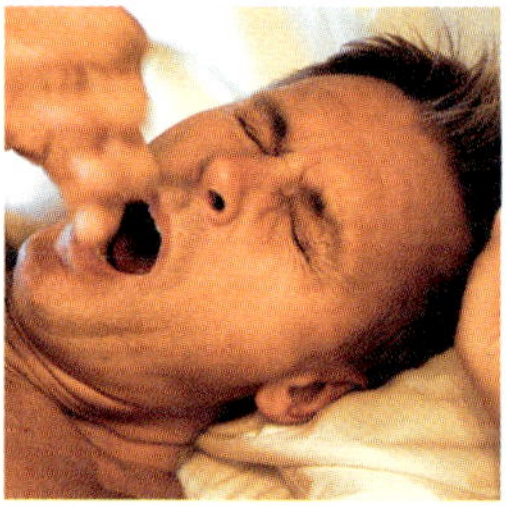